SCI

JAN 1 3 2012

D0116884

COMMANDER IN
CHIC

Also by Mikki Taylor

_Self-Seduction: Your Ultimate Path
to Inner and Outer Beauty_

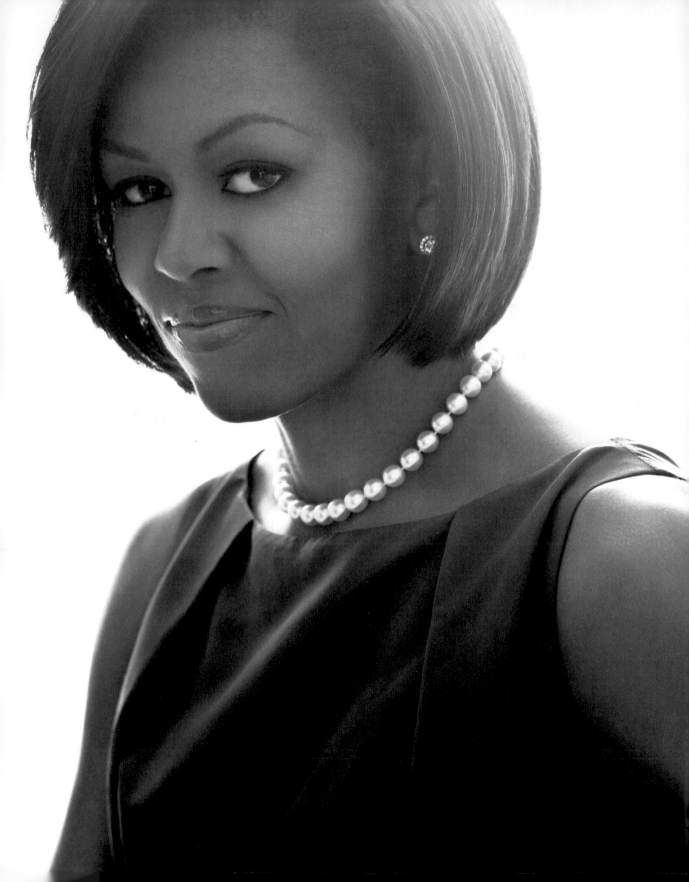

COMMANDER IN
CHIC

Every Woman's Guide to Managing
Her Style Like a First Lady

MIKKI TAYLOR

3 1336 08966 0949

ATRIA BOOKS

New York London Toronto Sydney New Delhi

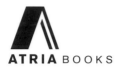

ATRIA BOOKS

A Division of Simon & Schuster, Inc.
1230 Avenue of the Americas
New York, NY 10020

Copyright © 2011 by Mikki Taylor

All rights reserved, including the right to reproduce this book or portions thereof in any form whatsoever. For information address Atria Books Subsidiary Rights Department, 1230 Avenue of the Americas, New York, NY 10020.

First Atria Books hardcover edition November 2011

ATRIA BOOKS and colophon are trademarks of Simon & Schuster, Inc.

For information about special discounts for bulk purchases, please contact Simon & Schuster Special Sales at 1-866-506-1949 or business@simonandschuster.com.

The Simon & Schuster Speakers Bureau can bring authors to your live event. For more information or to book an event, contact the Simon & Schuster Speakers Bureau at 1-866-248-3049 or visit our website at www.simonspeakers.com.

Designed by Jason Snyder

Manufactured in the United States of America

10 9 8 7 6 5 4 3 2 1

Library of Congress Cataloging-in-Publication Data

Taylor, Mikki.
Commander in chic : every woman's guide to managing her style like a first lady / Mikki Taylor.
p. cm.
1. Beauty, Personal. 2. Fashion. 3. Clothing and dress. 4. Obama, Michelle, 1964– I. Title.
RA778.T364 2011
646.7—dc23
2011016793

ISBN 978-1-4391-9672-4
ISBN 978-1-4391-9674-8 (ebook)

The information and advice presented in this book are not meant to substitute for the advice of your physician or other trained healthcare professionals. You are advised to consult with healthcare professionals with regard to all matters that may require medical attention or diagnosis and to check with a physician before administering or undertaking any course of treatment or diet.

To Mommy, my Commander in Chic forever,
with immeasurable love.
You are always with me in spirit.

CONTENTS

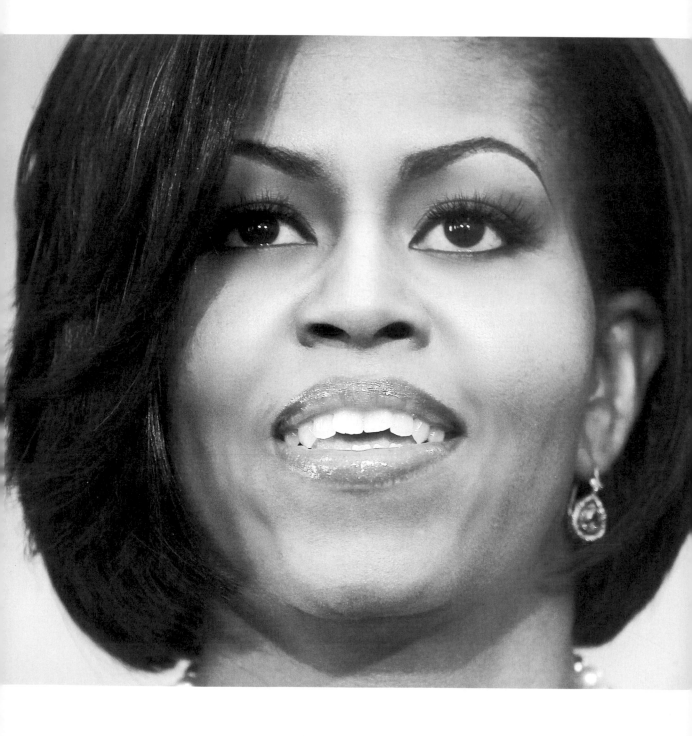

INTRODUCTION

Looking back, I never dreamed I'd see an African American woman as First Lady during my lifetime. It was always a vision in place for my children's future, an idea that would come to life in a time I wistfully spoke of as "someday." And yet there was no doubt in my mind the day I stepped into her home in Chicago for a cover shoot the summer before Barack Obama was elected to become the next president of the United States of America that "someday" had come and that I was looking at our soon-to-be First Lady, Michelle Obama. It was in the air, in her aura, and on the faces of the folks who passed by the house with a smile and quick toot of their horns as if having their "say-so" long before casting their vote.

It wasn't the first time I had worked with Mrs. O. We met in 2006 on a photo session that saw me directing her look for a power story in *Essence*. Now here I was sitting across from her at the dining room table discussing my vision for the cover—what she should wear, the hair, the makeup, the mood of the shoot, and so on. The conversation was flowing so easily; it was like I was talking to someone I'd known and loved for years. This time I was a little nervous, though, for I just felt like this would be the last time I'd be talking to her as the "senator's wife." Moments into the conversation, as I was admiring her ultra-chic dress, we both burst into laughs when she told me it was from H&M! At that point, I said to myself, "Okay, let it go girl. She's the real deal!" We decided on an elegant purple sheath for the cover and coordinating looks for Sasha and Malia and we were on. Of course, when the future Pres arrived home and proceeded to bring out his shirts for the shoot—asking *yours truly* which one should he wear—I had a truly comedic moment in that I was lost for words, and

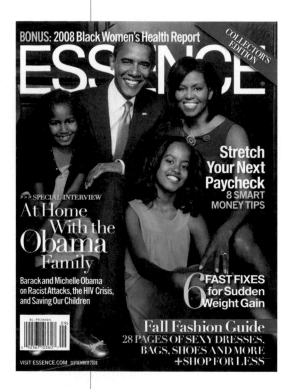

anyone who knows me is clear that I am *never* at a loss for words—especially not when it comes to style. But I lost all my composure chops that day and was totally "underwater" trying to give him an answer! He could have shown me a checkerboard shirt, and I would have said, "That's fabulous!" Nevertheless, I managed to find my voice and select a shirt for the "money shot" as we call it. My colleagues of course were in hysteria as they'd never seen Ms. Mikki loose her composure. That was one for the record, as they say.

Leaving the house that day I realized that one of the most fascinating attributes about Mrs. O is that she so gets it on every front. Her approach to life is deliberate across the board, and she's ever so clear in a world filled with confusion and ever-changing standards about the importance of setting your own. She's the woman for all seasons, who knows how to "do levels," as we say in the community, in that she knows how to look fabulous while being frugal, how to go from comfortably talking with the Queen of England to encouraging the youngins at Newark, New Jersey's, Maple Avenue School about the importance of eating

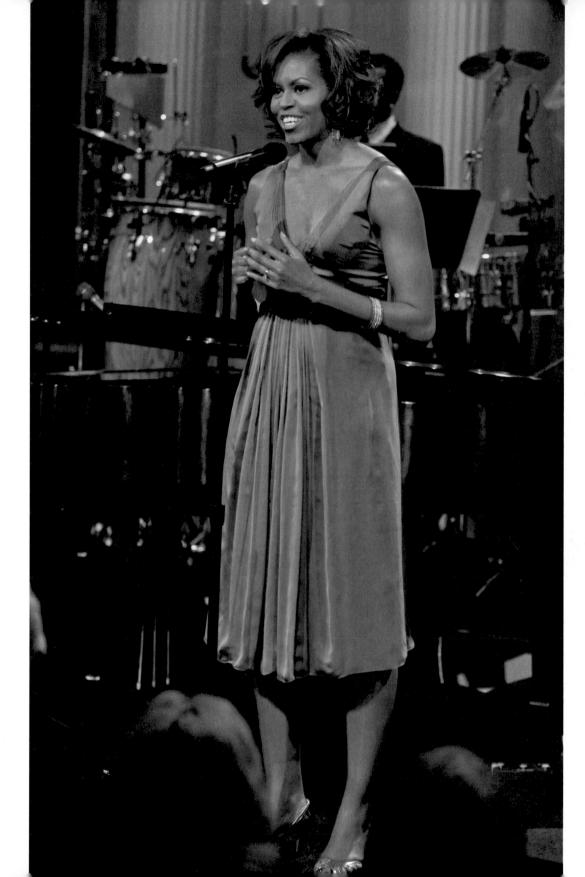

healthy. She's the sister-girl sprinting in Converse sneakers across the White House lawn by day who just as comfortably slips into a dazzling cocktail sheath by Kai Miller by night, welcoming Stevie Wonder to her home at 1600 Pennsylvania Avenue (see previous page). To say she's in full management of her own life and yet all the while looking out for the best for others is an understatement.

She has revolutionized our thinking about what's really key to *living*, not just going through the motions and being at our best in every way. For certain, she doesn't just have a full plate, she's balancing a platter: she's married to the most powerful man in the world, is a great mom, a beloved daughter, and a fab "Sis," all of which present a full set of responsibilities and cares of the heart. Yet by choice she's also focused on the wellness of the nation's children and the well-being of military families. There's not one of us who isn't moved by watching her step to purpose, day in and day out. We've long known her forerunners in our families and in the community as she's the sister we've always looked up to, the more-than-busy mom who still finds time to help others with passion and verve. She's the big sister who "never let them see her sweat," by staying focused on the duty at hand and all the while managing to keep a sharp eye on enjoying her life.

We've been waiting a long time for "Michelle Obama"—a true role model, not an icon—to come to life in the White House. This smart, savvy sister who looks like us, speaks like us, and brings a formidable determination to the table that's as tall and sure-footed as she is at nearly 5'11", walked in the door, ready to do the critical work. Her agenda is our agenda: that of taking back our health, canceling out obesity and therefore disease on *our* watch. It's dispelling that "angry Black woman" syndrome that folks at-large have tried to place on those of us who say what we mean and are affirmed enough to roll up our sleeves and place our hands on our hips while doing so. She's not angry, nor are we, just tired of "the way things are," as she told the women at a Las Vegas community center while on the campaign trail. Having embarked on what she herself has described as one of the best jobs in the world, she also sees her role as First Lady as an opportunity to help women transform their lives.

Living her life from the inside out is what has made Obama a woman to watch in every way. It's one reason why we're all captivated by that smart, chic fashion sensibility of hers that captures our attention every time she emerges—anywhere in the world. Because, as senior advisor Valerie Jerrett has said, "Michelle Obama is Michelle Obama's role model." In other words, she sets her own standards for what works for her. Through her role as First Lady and rock star brand, Obama has ushered in a period of optimism and purposeful style. She works American designers and retailers like a head of state! She wows us with newness, while remaining true to her style and what it means to be well dressed. She's also teaching us that you can be price conscious and look just as elegant and moneyed as if you had spent your wad. Michelle more than proves that you can have fun with fashion, wear what you love, dress powerfully, and yet not be bogged down by old rules that have nothing to do with how you want to live your life. She has established a signature style that works for her when it comes to fashion and beauty and loves working a "classic with a twist" theme that allows room for experimentation but is never off-track. At the end of the day, isn't that what we all yearn for? A signature style and a working wardrobe based on bankable pieces that allows one the kind of versatility where you never have to worry about what to wear? I say yearn no more: consider *Commander in Chic* as your personal style diary. From chapter to chapter, you'll find everything you need to know to possess great style—simply, effortlessly, and for keeps. Trends come

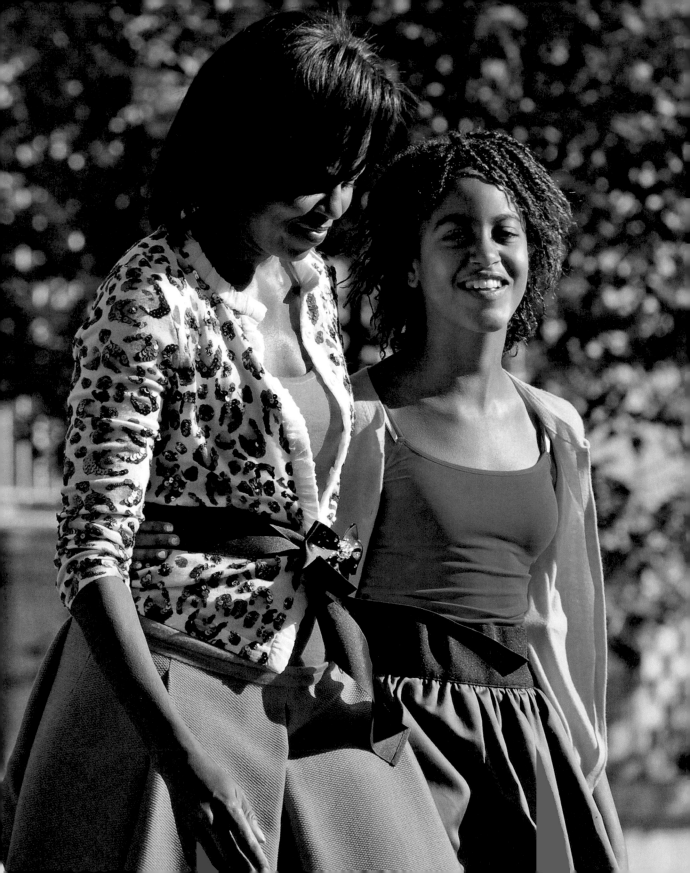

and go, but great style is forever "in." Besides, you're more than a season of someone else's style whims, so starting now, please don't take trends too seriously.

Beginning with chapter 1, you'll learn what to bank on and when to pass when it comes to establishing memorable style. You'll have your own personal checklist for those core pieces I deem "style essentials" for every great wardrobe—from a great cashmere cardi to "the little black dress" that takes you from day to night. I think every piece you buy should serve you on multiple occasions. I don't think you should ever buy a look for a single event unless it's your wedding—then you're allowed! In chapter 2 you'll learn how to determine your own dress code, shop smart, and always be well dressed. Speaking of shopping, you'll find the all-time checklist of fabulous resources from ultra-chic retailers to divine online destinations that will make shopping a pleasure once more. And when it comes to accessories, you'll not only gain insights on what to take from Obama's "it" list, but moreover what should be on your own, mileage-making list—and trust me—it's not about the most photographed shoe or bag, but rather those glam-slam picks that work and work without becoming dated.

But there's more to great style in this time of purpose than getting dressed. As Mrs. O demonstrates, *style* is really about how you see yourself from within and the care you in turn give yourself in light of recognizing your value. Watching Obama work it as a savvy working wife and mother who's carving out time from her busy life to self-nurture and invest in herself, to serve the nation and still sit down to dinner with her family, is more than motivating. And the fact that she has set a healthful agenda in the White House kitchen for years to come makes one say, We love you for it! Ditto for inspiring us all to move and exercise away disease and bring on wellness. In fact, chapter 4 will show you what you need to know to be healthy and fit at any age—from the types of exercise that you should be about by the decade to healthful eating for life. And while you're on the way to where you want to be, it will help you play up your best assets in style.

Being her most authentic self lies at the heart of Obama's seemingly effortless take on everything—from maintaining a workout routine that both keeps her tight and fit enough to travel the world with the president and yet live her own busy and fulfilled life to knowing herself well enough to close out the day at the appropriate hour and go to bed! We know full well the impact of burning the candle at both ends—stress, weight gain, and a checklist of adverse effects too daunting to mention. I know the pressure of trying to respond to the variety of responsibilities presented to us in this day and age. But once you read the daunting facts on our health and how we're inviting disease into our lives in chapter 4, you too will know when enough is enough. You may not get up at 4:30 to work out like Mrs. O, but you'll find your hour! I know I did. You'll also find that you love the value of juicing and choosing raw and healthy foods over processed, dead foods that take more than they give.

Now when it comes to your beauty, I've got you covered—from the best nude hues in makeup and modern, effortless techniques to how to gain and maintain healthy hair. With the product picks for healthy tresses to tips from Mrs. O's personal hairstylist Johnny Wright and versatile style options on the bob, you can't lose! When I began writing this book, the effort was no different than that of my former columns in *Essence*: it's all about moving us forward, whether through fab finds or fab news to take us to the next level. Like any great model or celebrity that I've worked with, Obama became a metaphorical muse for me. I love what I see every time I'm in her presence or watching her on the world's stage. It's all about the details—how she pairs "this" and "that," that radiant skin she possesses, that glossy head of hair, the grace she brings with her wherever she goes. Listen, we can't leave anything to chance when it comes to great style. In fact, I was so moved about this that the *last word* in this book speaks to us all about possessing great style from within, from clearing out the clutter in our lives to being the gatekeepers to our "sacred space"—our minds—so we can be our most striking selves.

So what's our "takeaway" in the era of Michelle Obama? That you must be determined to *own your life*, as this is your fascinating journey, and you owe it to yourself to be in charge! That you place a keen focus on living the life *you* desire so it doesn't elude you. In other words, don't live any part of it in the gray or leave any part of it to chance, or your richest desires will get away from you, and that's too great a price to pay. Don't waste a moment talking about it or dreaming of it—like Obama, possess it, *own* it. You know wish lists are for children. Women have checklists! So make sure you constantly self-edit by making those choices that affirm you without and within *all* of your endeavors and let go of anything that doesn't meet that criteria. And that means you've got to stay focused on what's important to you so you'll live *your* life as opposed to *acting* out the one someone else thinks you should live! That means you must have an intimate relationship with yourself and be self-nurturing and mentally aware.

If you look at Michelle's life, you'll see that she is on course because growing up she was encouraged to be so. The takeaway: don't settle. If you have a passionate goal, go for it. You may have gone to school to be a lawyer, but your yearning to fly could one day put you in the cockpit—so keep your mind's eye open. Make that self-discovery, and know that your desires are more than a notion. They could secretly be your passions, thresholds to your destiny. Why suppress them? You owe it to yourself to find out. To do so, you've got to learn to lovingly say "no" to things that keep you busy and often are a waste of your time and your gift (let alone your intelligence) so you can say yes to those things that are fulfilling and move you forward. It certainly means you have to let go of the pressures of what others might think if you're going to step out on faith; you can't use the hesitation. Obama lives in a fishbowl, and yet she's unmoved by the critics. We can certainly move on in our lives without being distracted by the opinions of others.

Obama clearly understands her worth and purpose and is motivating us to master our own lives with the same clear-cut assurance. We know this is essential to being the empowered women we are called to be. Through the Obama lens, we have seen that the most critical piece in life is to first glean what it takes to master "you"—to master your life—because if we're not owning our lives and celebrating our health and beauty, if we're not understanding our purpose, leading by example, and walking steady in the face of both challenge and success, then what are we doing in the vessels on loan

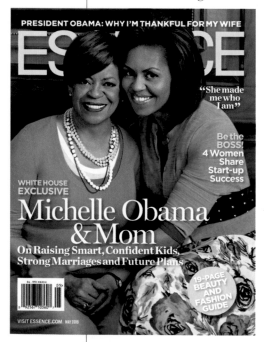

to us for such a time as this? Because life is not a dress rehearsal. This is it. The time of impact is now, so it really comes down to how well we're going spend it, and that's about making choices and seizing quality over quantity— something Obama is doing well. Quite frankly, I love her deliberate perspective, because I don't want to see us "do" more. We don't need another thing on the list; rather, I want to see us *be* more, and that's where purpose enters in. So be about doing the decisive work in your life in order to "live," not just exist.

As a mother, Obama's old-school values are enhancing the teachable moment, proving that everything *old* isn't antiquated and that ultimately raising wise and poised children has everything to do with teaching them love, temperance, and responsibility. As a businesswoman, she shows us that success is where preparation meets opportunity and that it's not only about reaching your goals, but also about wielding the power of influence from a motivating perspective—one that requires you to "lift as you climb," as the old adage goes.

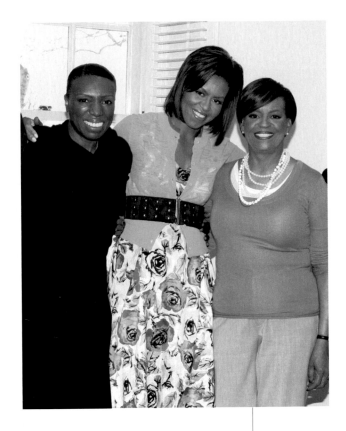

At the end of the day, style in the broad stroke is about being on purpose. It's about being comfortable in your skin and not following the trends but *setting* them. Finally, it's about being your most bold, empowered self and using that awareness to color your world—from your inner and outer beauty to your fashion sensibility, from the love that you share to the hand you lend in service to others. It's about showing up ready to stand and deliver and not only looking the part, but being just the woman for the opportunity at hand. That's what being a "commander in chic" is all about. And we, like Michelle Obama, are just the women to do so. Enough said.

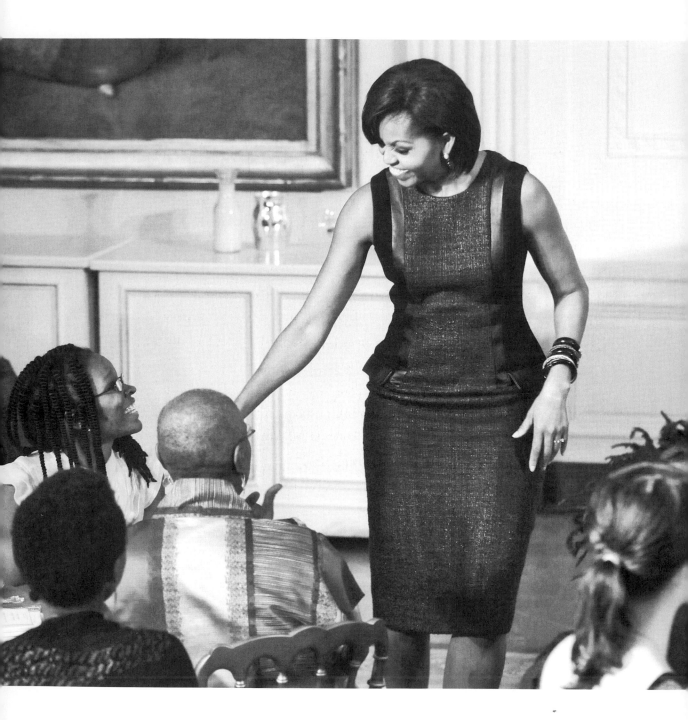

1

BANK ON IT!

From the moment she stepped on the world's stage, Michelle Obama became the iconic embodiment of "the teachable moment" on the subject of great style. She's setting the tone of the day for women, with her good works and with her "classic with a twist" style. When it comes to being well dressed, she follows her own rules for what works and what doesn't. In doing so she offers a new paradigm for every woman, raising the question of, what works for you? Not anyone else but you. In ushering a new era of style, we can see that color works for her, as does a great dress paired with a chic pair of flats. She has forever kicked to the curb the notion that First Ladies need to don a suit and proper heels to be taken seriously. Says who! What I know to be true is this: ever since the dawn of that coldest of inaugural days, Michelle Obama has been creating a new proverbial look book of bankable fashion for women around the world. Other notable women of style have graced the portals at 1600 Pennsylvania Avenue, but never has one come forth whose style is so bold, brilliant, and yet totally accessible. And it's a wardrobe that utterly works as it's chock full of the kind of essential go-to pieces that allow her to make those "repeat performances"—those looks that she works over and over again—with a fresh new twist every time. It's no wonder her bankable style has caused such a surge—from the cash register to the stock market—as she mixes couture with affordable retail brands that are available to millions. She's also made American fashion the "aspirational buy" (a style sensibility that everyone wants to work) just through her fearless approach to defining what it means to be smart and chic. She embraces new designers and brings a spirit of fun to what she wears. Maybe that too is the *vive la différence* she brings, in that she doesn't play the mystery game so embraced by others at the top of their style game. What you see is not only what you get with her, but also you can afford some of that, too! You can see the First Lady chatting it up with Jay Leno in a J.Crew look that you can buy online, and the next day *you* can take the same pieces and style them your own way. Her eye is not unlike that of a fashion editor who's constantly in "forecasting mode," and like the millions of African American women who color the world, she is a trendsetter—not a follower. In truth, we have always taken the so-called basics and given them distinction in such ways that we've quietly influenced the industry—from fashion designers who hired Black stylists to put their runway collections together to editors who hit the streets from Kingston, Jamaica, to Harlem's 125th Street to get hip to how we do it! Among her many strengths is her ability to take the basics and look sophisticated but not stuffy or old-fashioned. She's made cardis youthful, sheaths fresh, brought the spring coat back in. That's big for the millions of women who've never owned one or simply thought the trench coat was the end-all be-all. Our grandmothers and the millions of sisters hitting their closets or the nation's vintage shops could tell you a thing or two about the importance of having one. Though perennially classic, there is life beyond the trench coat! At a time when the casualization of America (which began with that great error of society known as "casual Friday") has almost wiped out sophistication, it's important that Obama is on the world's stage and having a "say-so" by bringing back sophistication. Her choices make getting dressed a real pleasure once more.

First Lady perks aside, with Michelle's style sense, there isn't a day when she'd ever have to worry about what to wear because she's built a timeless wardrobe that works around the clock and calendar. When you think about it, there isn't a woman in the world who doesn't want this same ease. It all revolves around core pieces with undeniable quality that keep one confidently well dressed.

MIKKI-ISMS

Do make a shopping list at the beginning of each season, filling in what you need first and foremost— especially anything that falls in the investment category—and shop accordingly so you're not all over the place buying clothing and never having anything to wear. Trust me—it happens more easily than you think. Impulse buys will turn your closet into a museum quicker than anything I know. There'll be much to admire—but getting dressed won't be worth the cost of admission!

STYLE ESSENTIALS

Mrs. O's inspiring wardrobe of ultra-chic go-to pieces reads like a who's who in fashion. While I wouldn't call it a formula, there are some investment essentials that have emerged, and they are such that any woman can take note of and make them her own. Here, at a glance, is your close-up on bankable buys:

The Cashmere Cardigan

Obama has replaced the once politically correct jacket that seemed to be the standard of a First Lady with smart, chic cardigans. She works this now staple piece over everything, from pencil skirts to sheaths, and at occasions that run the gamut from TV appearances to glittering White House receptions. Mrs. O has made this a signature piece and has them in what seems like a rainbow of hues. She dresses them up and down with assurance, but rarely matches them, as in a twinset.

Your takeaway: The jewel-neck cashmere cardigan is a great adaptor, always smart, forever chic. On today's retail landscape, you can purchase a great cashmere cardigan in all weights, shades, sizes, and prices; you can even take it up a notch simply by a change of buttons. All represent sound reasons why this piece is one to bank on.

A Great A-Line Shift or Fitted Sheath

The enduring allure of a sophisticated dress is never to be underestimated, as the "Obama style book" indicates through an array of fabrics and hues.

Your takeaway: A great dress requires little to no thought—you just step in and go! It doesn't get any easier than that, but the options are endless. You can change the character of the dress just by switching up your accessories, which makes it such a mileage maker. And be reassured that you can take it to the office and be just as polished and professional as your suited counterparts. As a solid investment, you should aim for several clean-cut dresses or one great silhouette in a range of colors that you love so you can turn them into a multiplicity of fabulous possibilities. Polish is what it's always about, yet you can have fun and style it forward with unexpected hues, pretty prints, and splendid fabrics—like a seasonless crepe, a fabulous bouclé—even a great brocade, which Mrs. O favors as well. You can also choose from a range of flattering necklines, from the classic V or jewel neck to a great boat neck, or an off-the-shoulder cut and beyond. You can also keep it simple or subtly embellished (I just love a dress that brings its own timeless ornamentation to the party!), and in the most womanly fabrics that "move" or "shape," you can't go wrong. And if buying off the rack doesn't give you a dream fit, a great tailor will.

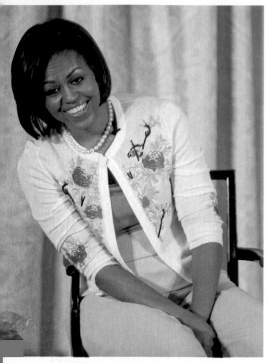

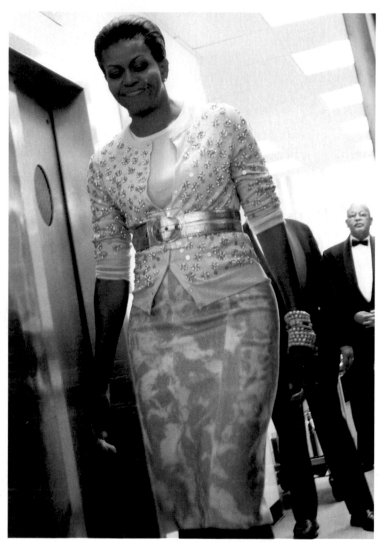

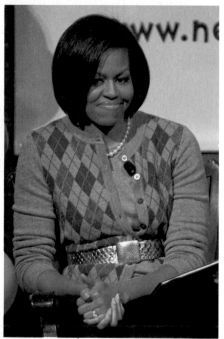

CARDI HOUR *The classic cardigan moves day-to-night and is perfect for a multiplicity of occasions—from casual weekends to evenings on the town. I love how Mrs. O works hers in a coolly confident array of hues, patterns, and textures. And whether the look is soigné and belted, clean and chic, or dazzling with embellishments, she never fails to look polished to perfection.*

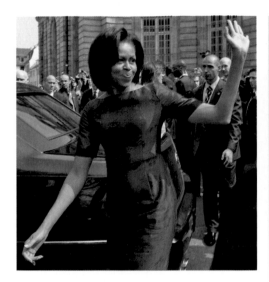

DRESS PARADE *In true Obama fashion, a great dress is such a style star! In particular, a fitted sheath or A-line shift stand the test of time. When well chosen, either delivers an immense amount of versatility, allowing you to change the persona and style it up or down to suit your desires. And, in the right fabrics, become a packable-friend that's always ready to go along for the ride!*

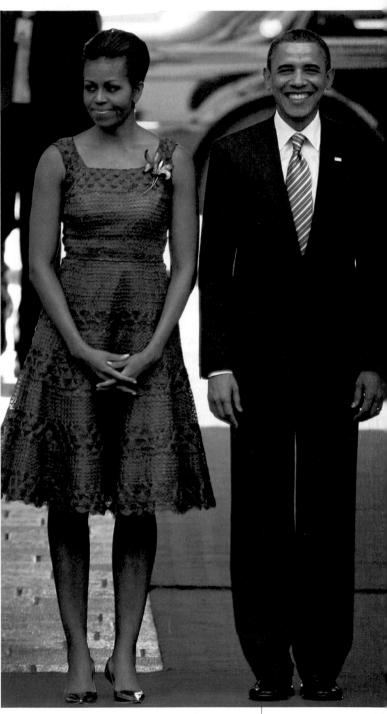

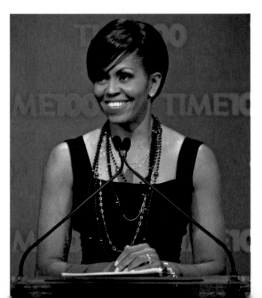

The Perfect Pencil Skirt

This beyond-classic piece is a sensational style setter. It too is quite adaptable, as Mrs. O demonstrates by working it as the great support piece that it is, pairing it with well with sweaters, blouses, and more.

Your takeaway: The pencil skirt can be styled to suit all of your well-dressed needs, especially in enduring fabrics. For certain you'll want to start your investment with the basic black find in, say, a lightweight gabardine. Know that a great fit—whether lightly tapered or one that just skims the body from waist to hem—will be worth the extra bucks. If you're ever in doubt, just do the "cost per wear" analogy in terms of how many times you'll work it and how that adds up, and it'll make you smile. Once your best basic is in place, add a few timeless colors and texture variations à la Obama and enjoy.

MIKKI-ISMS

What takes a pencil skirt from great to amazing? Why, a tailor, of course, and a fit-perfecting body shaper!

A Classic Duster Coat

Polished and always contemporary, the duster or buttonless coat pulls together a look instantly. Obama often belts hers or lets it swing over a great shift, turning it into a modern-day ensemble that goes from the White House to the church house and wherever Air Force One touches down!

Your takeaway: This is a real fashion investment, one that should be special yet simple enough to work over everything in your wardrobe. I have several that I've collected over the years in fabrics and hues that are anything but basic, yet they are versatile enough that I can work them with jeans, sheaths, trousers, and evening dresses. Choose a knee-length cut, an A-line silhouette, and a hue that you'll love every time you wear it.

MIKKI-ISMS

Who says you have to play "hue-solitaire" when it comes to a great duster coat? I say knock yourself out with great pattern-alia, but buy quality at all costs. Cheap prints are best on cosmetic bags!

PENCIL POWER *The pencil skirt is such an Obama trademark. Her wardrobe is pulsed by this power staple! Women of all ages can slip into this ultra-chic shape and rock, however, I say choose your pencil wisely. If you can run in it—it's too boxy! If you have to "tip"—be sure you can handle it. If you can walk like a lady—that's a sure bet!*

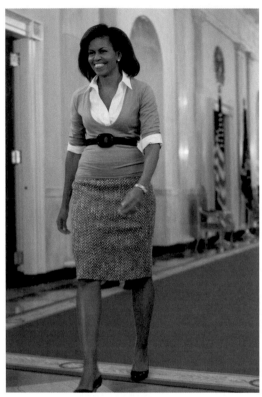

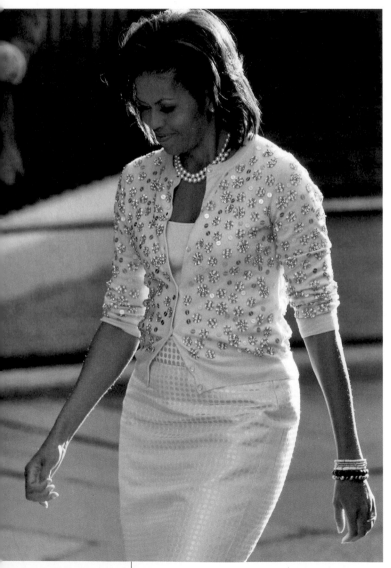

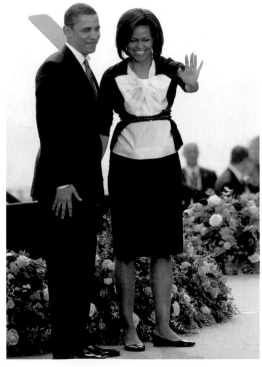

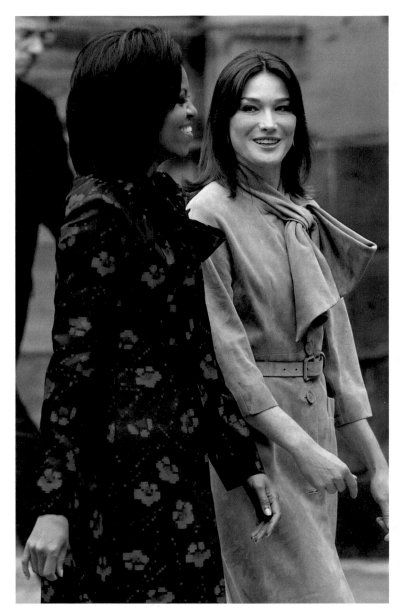

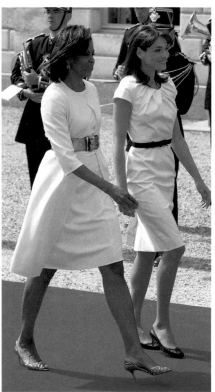

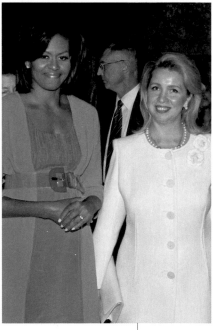

COAT CLASS The duster, or buttonless coat, is simply unstoppable! Obama always works hers with a heady dose of attitude and a bold extra—be it a waist-cinching belt or a fab brooch. Don't be left out in the cold, add this pick to your wardrobe and trust that you'll reach for it again and again!

Flared Pants

This elegant style staple with its soft, fluid lines works well under a myriad of pieces, keeping pace with a busy lifestyle that goes well beyond the nine-to-five day unlike any other pant "silho." The refined ease of a flared pant keeps Obama fashionably at ease no matter what's scheduled for the day ahead and really gives her a leg up on creative style possibilities as evidenced by how she pairs them with an array of pieces from jackets to dresses, as she did on a trip to Indonesia in November 2010. Even on those occasions when they're part of a suit, as in the case of her pale yellow Stephen Burrows showstopper, the look is graceful and chic as opposed to stiff, thanks to the inherent softness and movement this classy pant offers.

Your takeaway: Invest, invest, and invest, for you'll certainly want several great alternatives for repeated wear. Several years ago, I made the mistake of buying only one pair of a soft black crepe designer pant and much to my dismay, they sold out, and I was unable to get them or any quite like them again. Boy, was I sorry! So don't let this happen to you. Whether you choose those with a slim waistband or a good elastic waist that doesn't roll, look for quality fabrics like light crepes and tropical-weight woolens that won't lose their oomph at the dry cleaner's; stay on the lookout for great offerings in basic black and if you so desire, then fill in your color palette with navy, brown, gray, and winter white, which packs its own unique punch.

The Little Black Dress

This wardrobe powerhouse is like a good girlfriend—she never lets you down. The First Lady raises the style bar with her stunning array of ultra-sophisticated LBDs—from those that bare her toned arms like the Michael Kors sheath she wore for her official White House portrait to those that are three-quarter-sleeved and fitted, full, and flirty or soft and refined.

Your takeaway: Make the LBD your eternally chic pick, so you can pull it out again and again and look absolutely fabulous. Be it a minimalist sheath with a well-cut neckline and an impeccable fit that goes from the boardroom to a business dinner, a strapless wonder with a structured bodice and a pencil fit that sees you off to a black-tie reception, or a great timeless wrap number that allows you to dress it up or down, when you see a great black dress—pick it up. You'll love it forever. Always look for good fabrications and sophisticated cuts that range from simple to stunning; be determined to spend a little more for this forever-reliable piece and know that you'll never go wrong.

MIKKI-ISMS

Add zest to your best LBD with a conversation-worthy shoe in a knockout hue or a bold-hued, sexy matte lipstick!

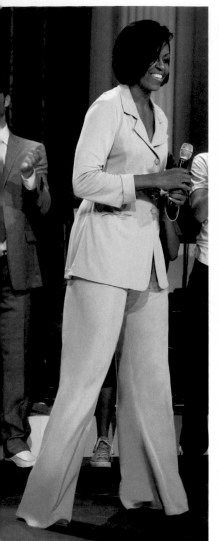

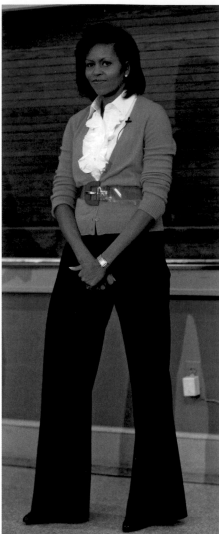

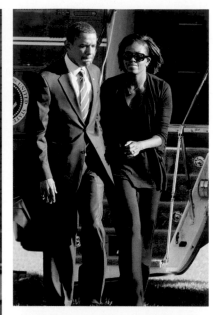

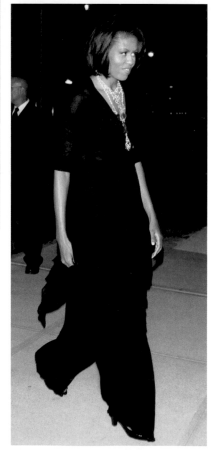

PANT LOGIC A great flared pant is eternally chic and classy. As evidenced here, Mrs. O's choices allow her to make the most mileage-making, modern pairings for her busy lifestyle. Think of them as an important player in your wardrobe and stock up. And remember: Always choose quality over quantity. But do buy quality in multiples!

Commander in Chic

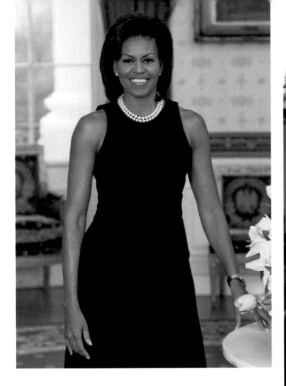

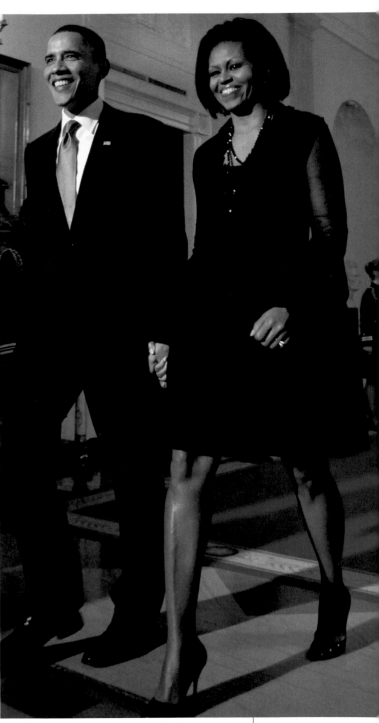

THE LBD FACTOR *The little black dress is a wardrobe mainstay. The First Lady has a seemingly endless collection of ultra-fab picks that satisfy her "code-chic" style ethic for every appearance. From clean and minimalist shapes to those that offer you maximum impact and great charm, think of the LBD as the smart, sophisticated option that it is and work!*

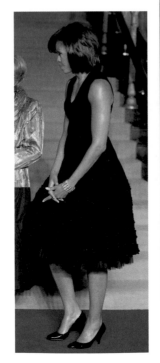

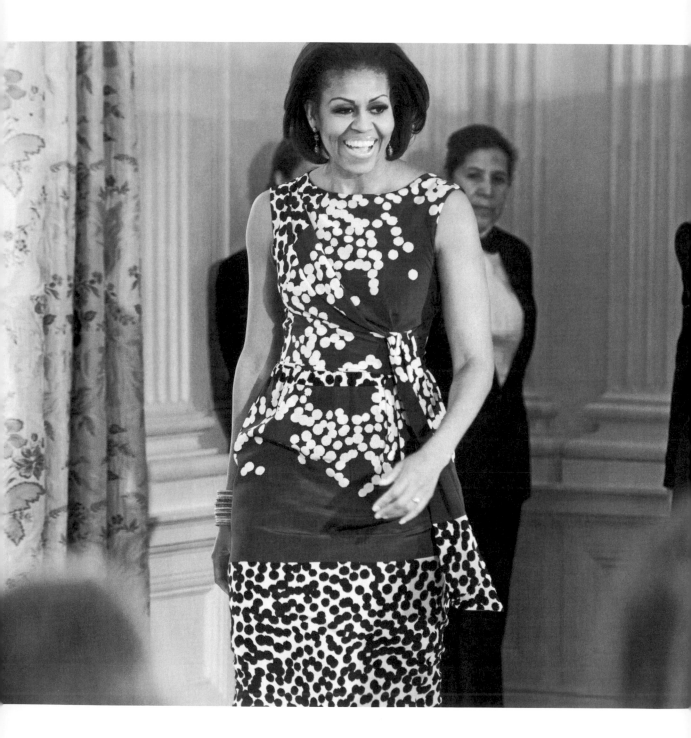

2

DRESS CODE

Michelle Obama plays a dazzling role as the nation's First Lady and looks every bit the part and more. What I find so inspirational as I travel this country speaking at various conferences and empowerment gatherings is that her trademark sense of style is captivating women everywhere. And clearly, as evidenced by her first two years in office, has also made her a modern-day muse for the nation's top fashion designers. They not only vie to dress her, but also have begun to incorporate her approach into their lines for a fashionable public desirous of working her succinct, purposeful look. Day in and day out, our dynamic sister projects a covetable style that's always chic, modern, and effortless and one that we all can buy into.

And yet, simple as this seems, there's clearly a deliberate point of view here. Just look at her passion for color, texture, and prints that she works with a cultural authenticity, serving up the most unexpected mixes, as she did at the Clinton Global Initiative dressed in a Moschino Cheap and Chic multipatterned chemise that featured hothouse flowers on top and a digital print on the bottom or working a gray and nude lace J.Crew top with a tiered floral-print skirt while skipping hopscotch in Mumbai (see pages 18 and 19). Undoubtedly, I see elements of our African ancestry and our distinctive take on fashion mixology throughout history reflected

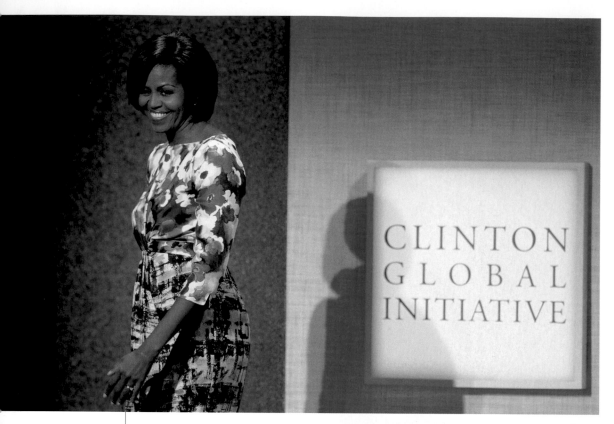

CLINTON
GLOBAL
INITIATIVE

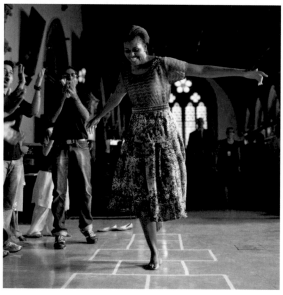

*Pattern, texture, and
unexpected pairings!
Mrs. O's confident
fashion sense allows
her to mix-it-up with
authority! She sets a new
kind of chic and places it
"on edge," in her day-to-
day, once again proving
one can have so much
fun with fashion and be
beyond well-dressed in
the process.*

Commander in Chic

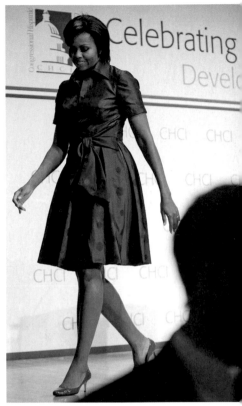

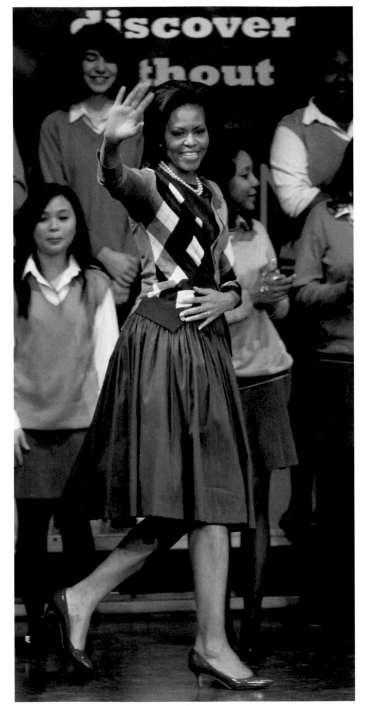

Obama's dress code is chic, fun, even playful at times, yet always grown-up and elegantly realized. Sharp selects and transformative accessories keep her look on style's fab track! I say, "Be inspired!"

throughout her dress code. Her pattern and texture combos—not to mention what could be considered a flamboyant use of color—these are our own, from Africa to the Carribean. Then there's her smart twists on the trends, where she takes new offerings and spins them her own way, whether by adding a belt or multiple brooches, or simply by marrying unexpected pieces, like the occasion where she worked a blue argyle cardigan by Junya Watanabe over a Peter Soronen shift and completed the look with a fashionably large strand of pearls (see previous page). Again, she never plays a look the way it comes down the runway—that's so not according to her MO! Analyzing her look, one can see that she definitely likes a touch of the eclectic, hence the fearless use of eye-catching accessories and baubles with presence. A lot like an African princess, no? She also makes what many women, especially those on the political front, would consider "a bold move," whereas she'll throw a curve to an otherwise classic look or ensemble by mixing in an unexpected element such as a punch of color by way of a shoe (like the cobalt blue pump she paired with Kevan Hall's bronze and navy shirt dress during a ceremony for Hispanic Heritage Month; see previous page) or an embellished cardigan that rocks as did the beaded J.Crew cardigan she wore during her early travels as First Lady to Europe, working all like only she can (see chapter 1, page 10).

MIKKI-ISMS

Don't ever be caught looking less than "code-chic." It's your reasonable duty!

In great style, according to Obama, there's also that heady dose of élan that sees her reworking "hi-res" (read highly visible) dresses in the public eye. My celeb sister-friends won't even break the rule of no-repeats! But Michelle is so focused and confident (as well as practical-minded) that style for her is really a state of being. So why wouldn't she continue to embrace the things that she loves? Given the state of the economy and the fact that there are much more important matters at hand, she sets a great example for us all when it comes to good taste and smart, forward thinking. It also sends the right message to our daughters and young sisters "on the climb" on how to separate your needs from your wants and value coining a look that works for keeps. The First Lady's wardrobe is composed of "keepers," pieces that she not only loves, but that also allow her to work a multiplicity of options using them as a base—in others words, she owns great mileage makers. And from where I sit, she does it well and with an unspoken belief that communicates it's not about the court of approval or necessarily about the trend for the new. For I see her going "back to the future" in many of her composed looks and speaking to those most ladylike elements. Rather, it's simply about great flair and how many ways you can spin it. Now there's a dress code that works. But that's just what lies on the surface. Behind every photo op and everything the First Lady does is a woman full of purpose who by example is encouraging us all to discover our own strengths, to know who we are, and to trust our distinction and fully enjoy the process of being ourselves. I can relate, for it's at the heart of what I do as an editor: communicate a message.

Every time I step into the studio, and no matter who I'm working with, be it an Oprah, a Mary J. Blige, an Iman, a Mo'Nique, or a Jada Pinkett-Smith, it's about communicating a look that expresses a distinct point of view. Ditto for those times when I'm "front row," viewing a designer's collection—my mind is spinning, deciphering a story that *I'll* want to tell. And that's the style secret that's at the heart of any great dress code or fashion message: a distinct point of view. It doesn't mean that I don't take chances, but when I do, I have a point of reference, a concept, and so the

MIKKI-ISMS

Please don't ever look as if you cared too much. A perennially chic sister is always modern, chic, and effortless in her appearance.

gamble is taken within a framework. The same thing holds true for Mrs. O. And though reporters around the world like to compare her to Jacqueline Kennedy, my take on it is this: sisters have *dressed* for ages and brought their own unique aesthetic to the fashion table—Obama is no exception. But as for First Ladies, I'd say that there hasn't been another standout since Jackie Kennedy (who, ironically, became the first Mrs. O). As for the millions of women who are informed by the ageless appeal of the Obama look and her Midas touch with fashion, I say develop your style with an appreciation for our rich history.

PRIMARY PURPOSE

Working color is a bold, fierce move that suggests passion, verve, and a strong sense of self. You have to have a positive attitude and confidence to push boundaries and heat up a look in an unpredictable way. The right hues can make you radiate, brighten your eyes, and be a standout. One thing's certain: color is never out of style in the hands of a great style setter. Mrs. O works color like an artist, with a palette of fresh, unexpected mixes and a *joie de vivre* that makes one smile. From jewel tones to highlighter brights, she has honed her use of color to a T, wearing eye-catching dresses, sophisticated separates, and electric accessories.

Tip It!

- Color is a mood lifter. A vivid hue can set the tone to "delight" and color your day or the evening ahead. With color you can **play it safe** by popping a bright over black; **push it forward** by working a set of complementary hues like citron and teal, or **push the envelope** by pairing two brights of equal intensities—like fuschia and orange.

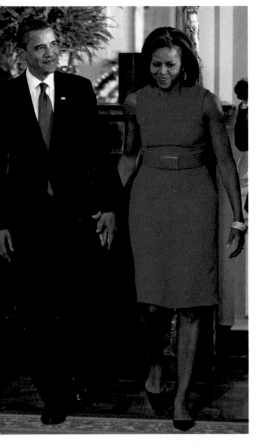

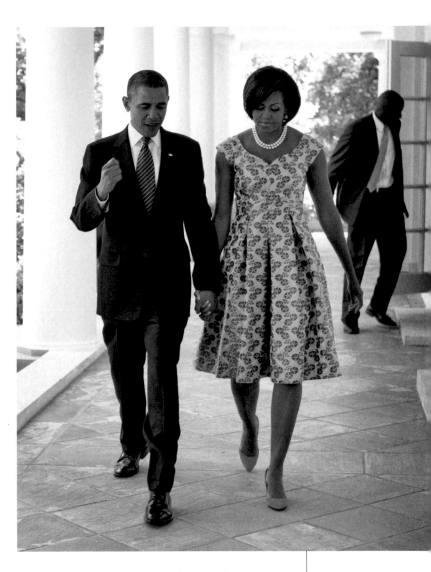

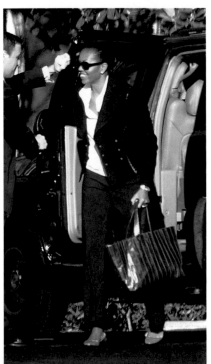

Obama kicks the charm of a ladylike sheath into "next" territory by pairing it with a pink kitten-heel pump. She serves lipstick-red against her chocolate skin with utter freshness. Black moves from basic to fashion forward with the edginess of bright blue flats and a racy teal tote.

- Be compelling by working a single striking hue, like a bold, lipstick-red sheath. A monochromatic use of color is always smart and sophisticated.

- When used strategically, color can play up the parts of your figure that you want to accentuate, so work it! Try pairing a chartreuse top with a navy pencil skirt—the bright top will illuminate your rich brown skin and play up your torso, while the dark skirt will instantly slim your lower half.

MIKKI-ISMS

Color? Why, color was made for a sister. Explore it like a fantasy you were meant to live: team teal, yellow, and violet. Toss on red and orange and kiss it with emerald! Engage orange and hot pink. We were meant to be seen. After all, the Creator dreamt us in color and scattered His chocolate sweets all over the world!

Commander in Chic

IT'S ALL IN THE MIX

Prints, pattern, and texture really add flair to a wardrobe and are a cinch to accessorize with a "less is more" approach. For certain, it takes panache to work them all simultaneously (as Mrs. O did at the 2010 Kennedy Center Honors where she pulled out all the stops in a dazzling floral sequined gown). Select one stunner in this category, call on it for big occasions, and opt for the staples that extend a wardrobe in your day-to-day, like a floral or leopard print top or a digitally patterned skirt, or even a great tweed shift with a subtle hint of shimmer that you'll wear year after year, updating it with new accessories as you go. One thing's certain: do mix. It's a contemporary style move. So whether you do so by wearing great shots of color-saturated florals or abstract prints, timeless geometric or cultural patterns or fresh, smart textures, work them in the chicest shapes.

Obama's choices always fall in line with her basic style aesthetic, whether via a great dress, well-thought-out separates, or strikingly fresh and simple evening wear.

MIKKI-ISMS

*Don't take **trends** too seriously. You're more than a "season of style whims"!*

Tip It!

- Impactful prints can give new life to timeless silhouettes without being trendy. When shopping, look for prints with distinction that you'll love forever. And if they say "notice me," so what? It's not a uniform!

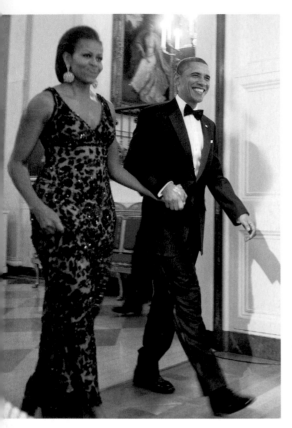

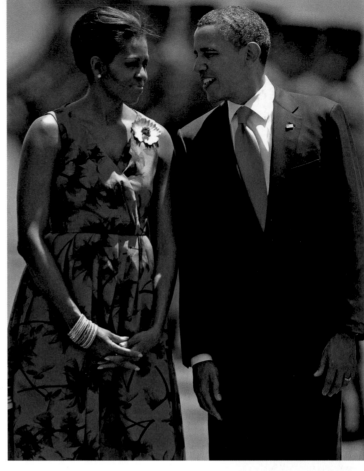

Mrs. O pulled out all the stops in this beaded Naeem Khan gown. A great printed frock—like this periwinkle blue wonder by designer Jason Wu— is not only striking and fresh, but also makes getting dressed a simply wonderful affair. A multipatterned top makes a statement all its own and takes a casual pair of slacks into ultra-chic territory.

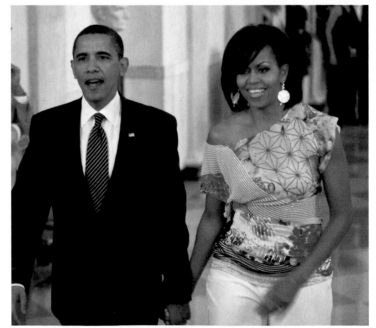

Commander in Chic

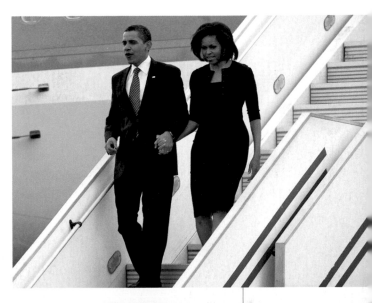

Mrs. O works this cropped black cardi day to night! Here it makes the scene by day over great separates. It appears again, giving fresh appeal to a smart black sheath. By night Obama popped it over a black-and-white satin empire dress for stepping out with Mr. O, and it was sublime.

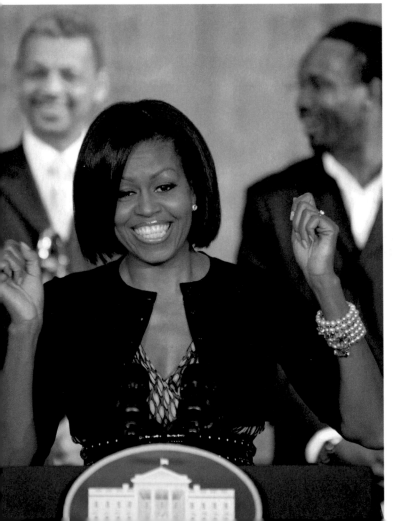

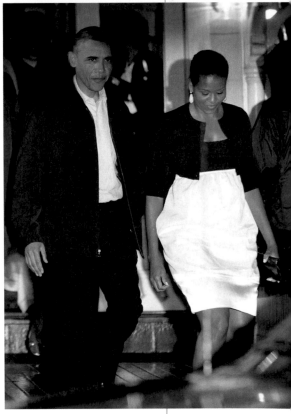

- Mixing and matching prints and textures on your own is a forward-thinking formula made simple by working them in the same range of hues.

- To quote an old adage, "Variety is the spice of life," and stunning patterns and textures in moneyed silhouettes never fail to add excitement to an otherwise basic look. Stay on the lookout for pencil skirts, sheaths, and charming blouses with pattern and/or texture pizzazz!

REPEAT PERFORMANCE

Great style is based on a wardrobe of signature pieces with an enduring chic that's both timeless and special. Unlike trendy pieces, these statement-making silhouettes reflecting one's personal style will always come out again and again, much to the delight of both the wearer and those she keeps company with! The distinctive pieces that beg for an "instant replay" are those that can be reinterpreted or reinvented with a fresh eye from season to season. Successfully working a style redux is about more than what you wear. It's really about how it makes you feel each time you wear it and how you want to turn it out time after time with a fresh beat.

The First Lady remixes separates that she loves with ease, but she's not daunted by repeating a great dress for an event. She just always makes certain to switch it up with a change of accessories or accent pieces like a great cardigan or a sublime jacket.

MIKKI-ISMS

Work a striking sense of style by playing the best pieces to new perfection.

MIKKI-ISMS

Some people say, "Never let them see you sweat."
I say look your most fabulous under
pressure *and have a good laugh while you*
keep them guessing!

Tip It!

- Be on the lookout for pieces that you can work in different ways and that are easily updated. Don't forego that piece that's simply to die for—just know when to play it.

- One of the joys of a great wardrobe is the ability to wear what you love again and again. A well-rounded assortment of super accessories will give you the mileage you need to bring change to any and all the pieces you love again and again.

- Remember, your goal is to dress in a way that conveys great personal style, and if ever there's a cause for a "repeat performance," that's one that counts.

MIKKI-ISMS

Do make sure every piece you buy
will serve you on multiple occasions.
Never buy a look for a single event unless it's
your wedding *—then you're allowed!*

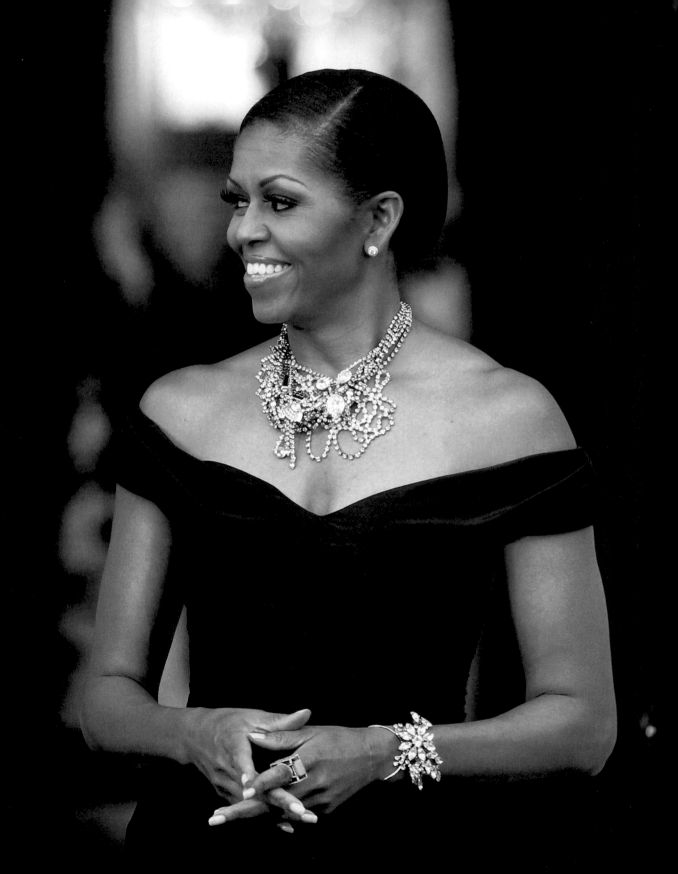

3

BOLD EXTRAS

To say Michelle Obama loves accessories is an understatement. She has revived them singlehandedly! On the campaign trail, Obama put accessories in the spotlight, from the most amazing brooches and power pearls to waist-cinching belts, kitten heels, and chic flats. On Inauguration Day she stepped into the spotlight, showcasing both her passion for color and love for turning up the volume on classic accessories. She wore a pair of unexpected green gloves with matching pumps. Now, as evidenced by over two years in the spotlight, she *works* accessories and uses them to play up her keen sense of style and give new dimension to being well dressed. Among her faves are her Azzedine Alaïa belts, her conversation-worthy brooches by Erickson Beamon, and piles of pearls in all sizes imaginable. She has such a great eye for working an eclectic mix when it comes to accessories that she's even shown her mother how to successfully layer necklaces to make a statement. I fondly remember her on the May 2009 cover shoot for *Essence* at the White House adjusting Mrs. Robinson's necklaces so they were layered just so (see Introduction, page XX). Obama's knack of styling with bold accents conveys the confidence she possesses about herself every step of the way. In truth, this is an area where how you see yourself really impacts the results. It's why one fuller-figured woman can wear belts so well and why another one shies away from them fearing she's too large to pull it off. They may be the same size but feel differently because accessories also say a lot about your emotions. Again, it's how you see yourself and whether or not you are striding—as Obama is—on the path of self-discovery. Accessories form the core of your personal style and convey the image you wish to project. Mrs. O uses them to define everything she wears and make it her own. This clear sense of direction allows her to narrow her choices of accessories and work them like an editor. She's so confident in her selections that she can work a bow on a floral Thakoon dress, pop a vivid blue pump with an inky deep chemise, or creatively turn an inexpensive dress into a moneyed look just by switching out the belt it came with and replacing it with one of her designer faves. She so knows when to drop a little cash on those "forever pieces" as well as when to play throwaway chic and pick up those "just because I love it items" that add fun and pizzazz at noncommittal prices. And from what I've seen, there's a euphoria that she gets from fearlessly "mixing it up" with accessories unlike anyone I've known—and I know the style mavens, from celebs to fashion stylists.

What I know for sure is that accessories are a passion worth indulging as they are the tools of self-expression. They also add great mileage to your wardrobe and carry a look through from season to season, day to night, fun to serious and more. One wonders if Mrs. O knew this from the start, as word has it that she bought her first Coach bag with her earnings as a babysitter!

MIKKI-ISMS

Do mix the best accessories— e.g., bracelets or necklaces—but please avoid what I call "the Xmas tree" syndrome. Choose your cluster wisely. Know when enough is enough. "It's not all ashore that's going ashore!"

32 | *Commander in Chic*

OBAMA'S "IT LIST" (PAGE 1)

If I could attach a motto to Obama's accessory style sensibility it would be this: "Keep it chic and fresh." The "objects of desire" that form her signature looks run the gamut from designer to bridge, from the essential "pops of color" to basic black. Many are embellished and some simply understated and sublime. What they all have in common: they reflect her flair for great style, at any price. Here's a look at what's in the mix of her essential accessory wardrobe, how they set the tone for her look, and why they say "must-have."

Brooches

The Style Maker. Mrs. O loves a great brooch, but don't pin her to any one look. She serves up an eclectic mix of buds, bows, bees, and more.

The Look. Bold, whimsical, aspirational; worked fearlessly on sheaths, jackets, and cardis, often in multiples.

The Message. Demonstrates a surefire way to add personal style, texture, and color to any look.

Pearls

The Style Maker. The First Lady plays them well—from the classic single and double strands to those that are big, bold, and fashion-forward.

The Look. From clean and ladylike to luxe, layered, and fashionably forward; worn at the neck as well as on her wrists; used as a signature staple that adds polish and interest to anything she wears.

The Message. Trends come and go, but pearls remain forever "in."

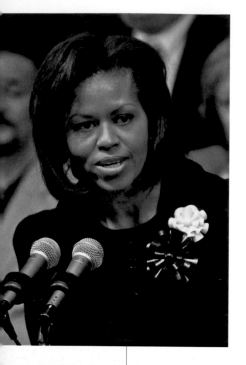

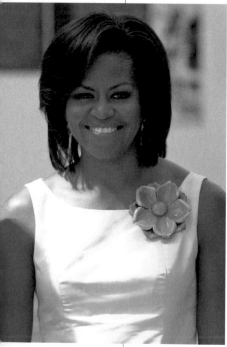

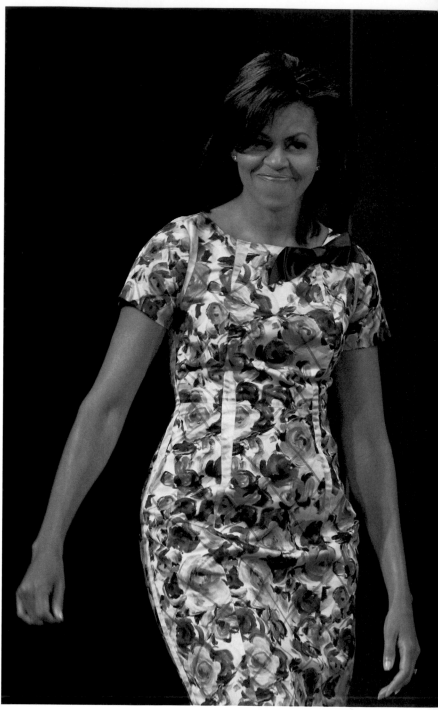

Commander in Chic

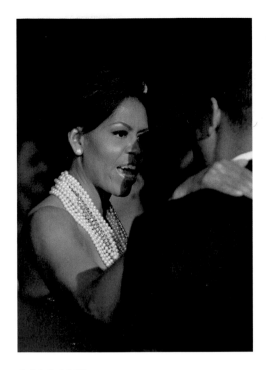

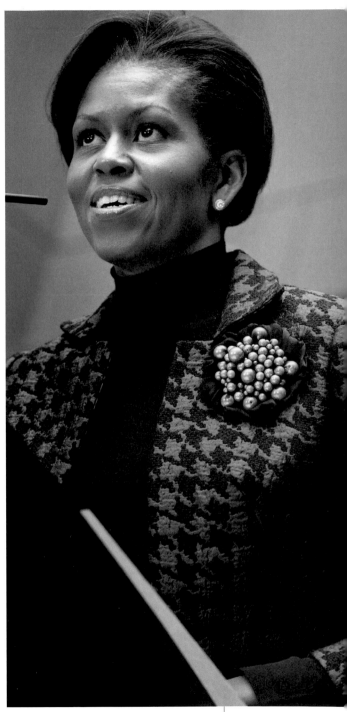

OPPOSITE

Obama wears brooches her way. Here she mixes it up in black and white. Only Michelle could pull off adding a bow to Thakoon's floral print sheath! The First Lady adds a whimsical touch to a serious sheath with a pop of color.

ABOVE AND RIGHT

Obama embraces the timeless elegance of pearls. A bold pearl brooch says it all. True to her "classic with a twist" style, Mrs. O works a stunning multistrand necklace of pearls and crystals by Tom Binns to perfection.

Earrings

The Style Maker. Obama mixes it up, working studs, hoops, dainty drops, and "chandeliers" with equal aplomb.

The Look. Impactful! Always lends just the right touch of elegance whether she's working a sheath or a dazzling gown.

The Message. Ear this: It's always about the right finishing touch.

Bracelets

The Style Maker. From delicate bangles to cuffs that dazzle, Mrs. O goes from chic, simple "stacks" to cuffs that make an impression.

The Look. In a word, *charming*. This Lady of Style often stacks an array of darling bangles or floats them in between understated cuffs.

The Message. If not wearing a great signature timepiece or a ring with presence, do accent your arms with something fabulous.

Belts

The Style Maker. Aside from pearls, belts have become the First Lady's style centerpiece, adding texture, color, fashion, and function to a great wardrobe. She's also quite adept at adding wattage and a moneyed look to inexpensive finds by switching out the accompanying belt for one of her designer faves.

The Look. Obama cinches a look with her now-signature Azzedine Alaïa belts, but also works savvy skins, high-shine patents, bold sashes, and metallicized wonders over and over with newness every time.

The Message. The right belt not only pulls a look together, but also makes it a standout in a cinch; a keen awareness of one's wardrobe needs and style sensibility are what should direct your choices.

Pumps and Flats

The Style Maker. When it comes to stepping into the eyes of the world, Mrs. O takes care of business in footwear that reflects her flair for fashion and passion for the new, the classic, and the comfortable.

The Look. A smart, chic balancing act—from a kitten-heel revival in all textures and hues to lots of gamine-style flats with toe cleavage and great peep-toe pumps.

The Message. Keep it fresh and unexpected, but never go to such heights that you sacrifice comfort for style.

MIKKI-ISMS

Calling all working girls: do
leave your "sneaks" for the gym.
Work a pair of elegant flats instead
when lowering your heels on the commute
to and from work.

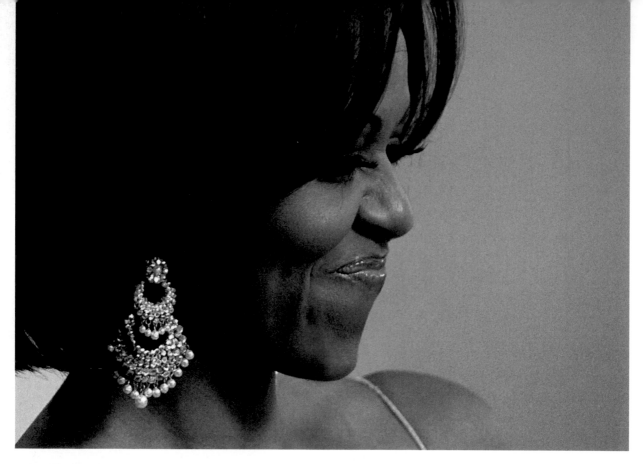

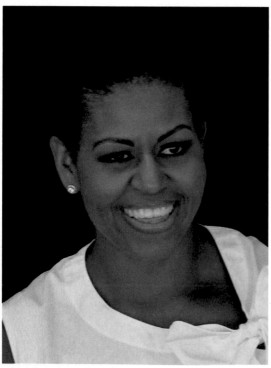

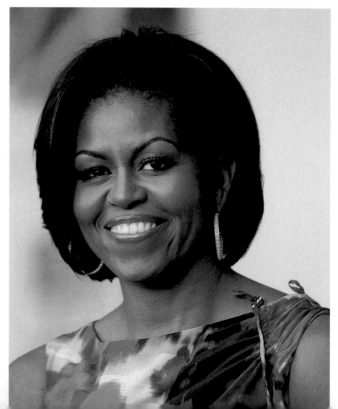

OPPOSITE

Dramatic occasions call for a bold statement, and the First Lady brings it as shown here in a pair of dynamic "drops" by Miriam Haskell. Colorful hoops lend a punch to this classic sheath. A pair of studs are Obama's "go with everything" style staple.

THIS PAGE

Obama loves to "bare arms," and this impeccable stack of white and gold bangles and cuffs is a fab way to do so! An eclectic mix of bangles and pearls by Alexis Bittar in a singular hue looks exceptionally rich. This exotic stoned cuff lends maximum impact to Mrs. O's clean style statement.

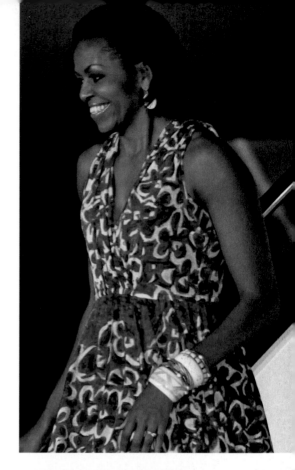

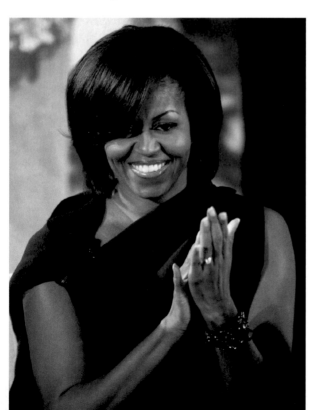

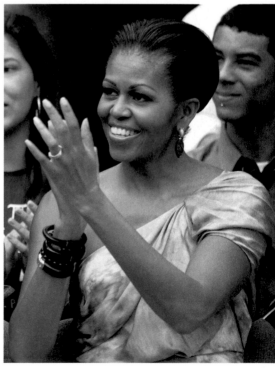

HAIL TO THE CHIC: TIMELESS ACCENTS ON STYLE — YOUR BEST BETS

Dressing well is about choosing the smartest accessories to boost your wardrobe mileage and make your every style move a fab, effortless experience. Contrary to what one thinks, it's not the "it" bag or the most photographed shoe that builds a successful collection, since they get dated pretty fast, but rather it's those glam-slam picks that work and work and thus are always "in." The well-dressed-and-in-the-know realize that at times it's about reimagining the tried-and-true and lending a dash of creativity that's uniquely yours, like changing the brown leather strap on your timeless watch to one in a chic orange or green snakeskin for a pop of color. Other times, it's about choosing a fresh, statement-making piece that stands alone, and before you know it, goes on to become *your* signature, because it's really about how well you wear a look as opposed to it wearing you. Finally—and surprising as it may seem—when it comes to nailing great finds, it's more about your eye and sense of style than it is your budget. My dear friend Pamela Macklin, wardrobe director to a number of style-setting celebs and high-profile women, has taught me this over and over again when it comes to accessories. My wallet and my bank account are much better off for it! Again, it's about having an eye for what works and not needing the so-called confidence of a high price tag to convince you that it does. *You*—not the cost or the shopping destination—are the reason why a great accessory works, so collect pieces that have what the French call a *je ne sais quoi* (read: something that cannot be

MIKKI-ISMS

When in doubt, always choose jewelry that **oozes sophistication.** *With picks like these, you'll never go wrong.*

adequately described or expressed, or, as I like to say, "beyond fabulous") that both excites you and stands the test of time. Here, then, is a look at what should be on your list of "look like a million" must-haves.

Pearls. Whether real or the most fabulous fakes your money can buy, as you can count on them to add polish to any look, from jeans and a tee, to a great sheath. When shopping, do mix it up and go beyond the hue of tradition. I have pearls in black, gray, and ivory that I wouldn't trade for the world. Don't tell my husband, but the classic white strand he had made for me comes out to play the least! Chalk it up to a fashion thing.

Diamond Studs. Real or cubic zirconia, as this sparkling addition makes a style statement day to night.

Hoops. Do yourself a favor and just buy the basics, a classic pair in silver and a pair in gold—the thinner the better—and let your imagination fly! I picked up a weightless pair in Cancun (a great shopping destination for fine jewelry, as is St. Thomas) several years ago, and I love them to this day.

A Cuff. Opt for one wide, go-with-everything cuff in gold or silver. It's a finishing touch that adds richness to most any look. I have individual cuffs that I've collected over the years—both simple and adorned—and they never fail to amuse me, while lending that certain something to anything I wear them with. Right now, I'm looking for a matching pair to wear '60s style—into the night!

A Cocktail Ring. This oversize addition is a glam slam, especially in the form of a single bold stone. Think of it as the exclamation point to a look and be expressive.

Classic Bands or a Trinity Band. You can't beat a great collection of bands that can be stacked to make a personal statement or a timeless

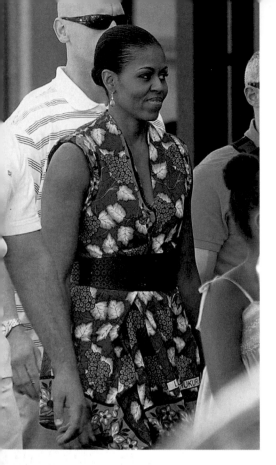

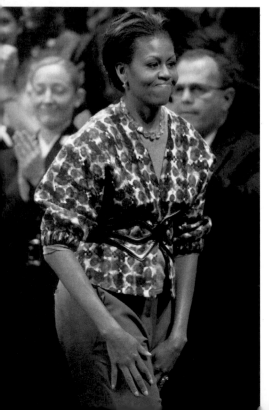

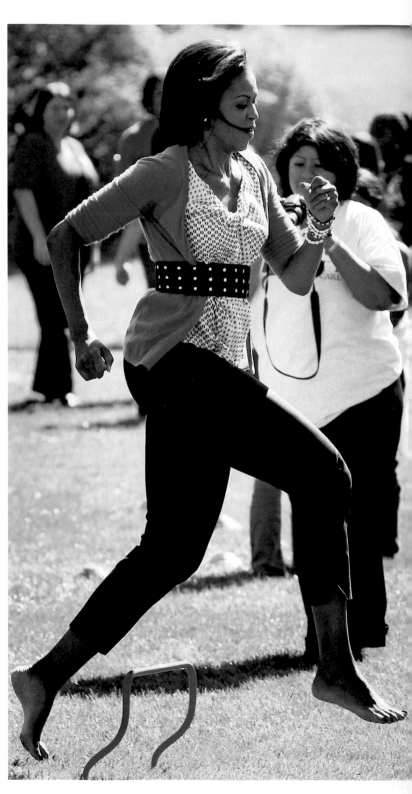

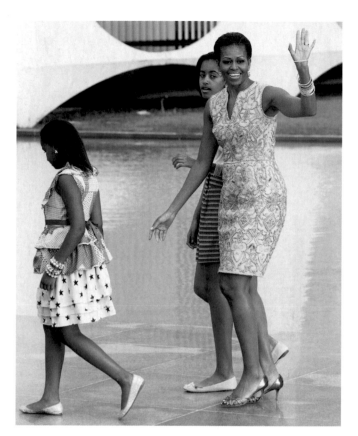

OPPOSITE

Michelle plays shape and texture to the max as in the case of these wide jet cinchers. The belt is a centerpiece: it defines, adds flair, and draws attention to Mrs. O's well-defined waistline. Even at play, the First Lady kicks it up a notch—here with her favorite Azzedine Alaïa belt.

THIS PAGE

Metallic peep toes, especially in a warm, skin-friendly hue, look elegant day to night. Gamine flats in a brilliant hue amp up Mrs. O's cool Tracy Reese sheath while keeping to her chic style sensibility. Obama clearly knows when it comes to footwear, "low" can have just as much impact as a stiletto, as evidenced by these fab peau de soie *kitten heels.*

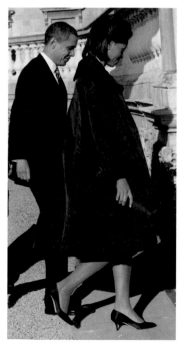

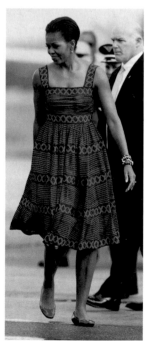

trinity band—both evoke a richness that lends character to anything you pair them with.

Gloves. Elbow and opera length; spring for a leather glove with a silk or cashmere lining or even those unlined (it's all about the quality of the leather), and a matte jersey for evening. Selections like these will work well with all the three-quarter-sleeved silhouettes that are here to stay, as well as with sleeveless sheaths and gowns. To me, the process of donning a pair of gloves is such an elegant experience. It's really too bad that a number of the great European glove houses have closed. I remember the first time I was properly fitted for a fine pair of gloves like yesterday. It was in Paris many years ago at a tiny shop where the city's fashionable women made their purchases. There, one would sit at the counter and lean over just so as Madame would stretch and fit your gloves to every finger. Watching them come out of the many cases, as thin as a sheet of paper—so much so that there was a special rod that was used to open up the fingers for the very first time—was absolutely fascinating. A simple "voilà!" and you knew she was satisfied and you were purchasing a pair of gloves that fit so well one would think they were custom made—not a bulge or a ripple in sight. Ah, the days of formality.

Brooches. From vintage finds to modern-day interpretations, from the bejeweled and the bold to the floral and utterly feminine—it's about "pinning on your imagination!," as my friend Macklin says.

A Luxe Scarf. A timeless, conversation-worthy silk scarf that can be worn at the neck, nonchalantly tied on a satchel, or wrapped around your head and paired with great hoops for a glamorous look unto itself is a wardrobe mainstay.

A Pashmina. In a soft, muted hue—it's your most polished coverup when the invitation reads "Black Tie."

Commander in Chic

A Classic Timepiece. A great investment—one that that adds character to any look and helps you "keep it moving!" I have a basic leather-strap timepiece, an old Tiffany classic that I've been working for years that allows me to play it fashion-forward or classic just by the switch of a band. I also have a great gold watch that becomes a piece of jewelry and works around the clock. It also layers well with a charm bracelet or a neat stack of gold or enamel bangles.

Sunglasses. A large, investment-worthy pair of dark shades with UV protection and a great case to protect them in are essential. "Shaders" are a trademark accessory that not only enhance your style (Mr. and Mrs. O rock them well!), convey glamour and chic-dom to the nines, but protect against the sun's damaging rays and the resulting fine lines. Need I say more?

A Transitional Clutch. This classic, in leather or patent, works overtime and never fails to look chic and elegant; one style caveat: the simpler the better, skip adornments and trendy detailing.

A Medium Satchel. Both polished and practical, this first-class buy is sharp, roomy, and just the day bag any accomplished sister should be swinging. Invest well as this one is repeatedly at your side and it should represent.

A Multitasking Shopper or Carryall. To tote all your needs in style without looking as though you're hauling around the "kitchen sink." Again, this is another investment piece that marries fashion and function, so make sure it's a quality buy but not a bore. It should be as chic as you are, work well solo or in conjunction with your clutches, and serve as your multitasker on the weekend and beyond.

MIKKI-ISMS

When heading to dinner after work, never tuck into a restaurant looking like a bag lady. Always carry a clutch and a fashionable tote or shopper that can be checked.

A Classy Flat or Skimmer. Easy, chic, and always appropriate, wear them with everything, from a great pencil skirt to a flirty dress that moves (channel Michelle Obama in that great Tracy Feith dress she works again and again) or jeans and more. One proviso: if you find a pair that you love, buy more in a few hues. You won't regret it!

A Pump with a Purpose. A great pump is the workhorse of your wardrobe—it needs to be all-purpose, have purpose, preferably have a low cleavage, and be well maintained.

Metallic Evening Sandal. A dazzling touch to your shoe collection that works across the board—from the prettiest cocktail dresses and gowns to the hippest jeans.

Black **Peau de Soie** *Pump.* The transforming power of a sharp silk pump in your wardrobe isn't to be underestimated—it's the elegant answer to all those great LBDs in your closet in that it will move them right into the night.

MIKKI-ISMS

No matter your budget, always wear **conversation-worthy** *shoes!*

4

GO FIGURE!

Much has been said about Michelle Obama's official White House portrait and how she's not afraid to bare her arms. Mrs. O is in such great shape that anything she wears conveys as much—from those long, lean, and beautifully sculpted arms and tight abs, right down to her well-toned legs. The First Lady sends a distinct message of confidence, one that encourages us all to be at our physical best. However, not to be misread, Obama is about more than great assets. She is about the business of owning the state of her health and well-being and encouraging others to do the same. That's true empowerment. As part of her strategy to be at *her* best, Obama makes maintaining her health an inner and outer pursuit, being mindful of what she eats and how much exercise she gets. Her old-school diligence is motivating at a time when surgical styling and quick-fix trendy diets are at an all-time high. She is one of our best examples of a person who honors her temple. She has an incredibly full schedule to balance, albeit with support. But she makes time to work out—with the president, no less—as well as plant a kitchen garden, launch a national campaign to tackle our obesity problem, and, especially, improve nutrition for the nation's children.

Manning the power seat when it comes to health and wellness is a position in which we must all be actively engaged. We can no more take our eyes off the road of our well-being than we could if we were behind the wheels of a car. I think tending our bodies with a keen awareness is vital to a future we want to have and a present we can enjoy. The fact that we can look absolutely gorgeous and dress to celebrate ourselves is just icing on the cake of good living. However, in this most celebratory moment in our history, the facts on our health aren't pretty. Here's the close-up on *some* of our greatest health challenges.

Heart disease is the number-one killer of African American women. Our smoking, high blood pressure, high cholesterol, diabetes, physical inactivity, being overweight or obese as well as having a family history of cardiovascular disease contribute to the high statistics. According to the American Heart Association, 44 percent of Black women have some form of heart disease. Another known fact: the risk of heart disease *increases* with physical inactivity and poor eating habits.

High blood pressure affects African Americans more than any other group in the country. Also called hypertension, high blood pressure increases one's risk of heart disease, stroke, and congestive heart failure. Forty-three percent of non-Hispanic African American women age twenty and older have hypertension.

High cholesterol affects nearly half of all African American women. Our diet tends to be too high in fat from animal foods, dairy products, and packaged as well as processed foods, and far too low in fiber from fruits, vegetables, and whole grains. Fifty-five percent of Black women are physically inactive, which also contributes to our high cholesterol scores.

Strokes occur when cholesterol, or plaque, build up in the arteries and block normal blood flow to the brain. A stroke can result in full or partial loss of movement, or speech, or cognitive function. Strokes can be fatal. The condition also increases the risk for heart disease and atherosclerosis, which are both risk factors for a stroke. About 42 percent of Black women have high or borderline high total cholesterol levels. African Americans age sixty-five and younger are more than twice as likely to have a stroke compared with Caucasians.

Diabetes affects nearly 15 percent of Black women age twenty and older. As we age, our risk of developing diabetes increases. It is estimated that nearly 50 percent of Black females born in the year 2000 and beyond will likely develop Type 2 diabetes in their lifetime. Among the factors that put us at risk are simply being overweight, having high blood pressure, high cholesterol, and lack of exercise. Among the many health problems associated with diabetes are: heart attack, stroke, amputations, blindness, kidney failures, skin complications, as well as both tooth and gum disease.

> ## MIKKI-ISMS
>
> *Don't be a "diet maven"— eat healthy for life. Being trim and fabulous should never be a temporary occurrence— you deserve better. Own it!*

Obesity disproportionately affects us, causing African American women to have the highest rates in the United States. Seventy-seven percent of obese women twenty years of age and older are African American. Being overweight or obese negatively impacts our health and is a factor in every form of disease listed above.

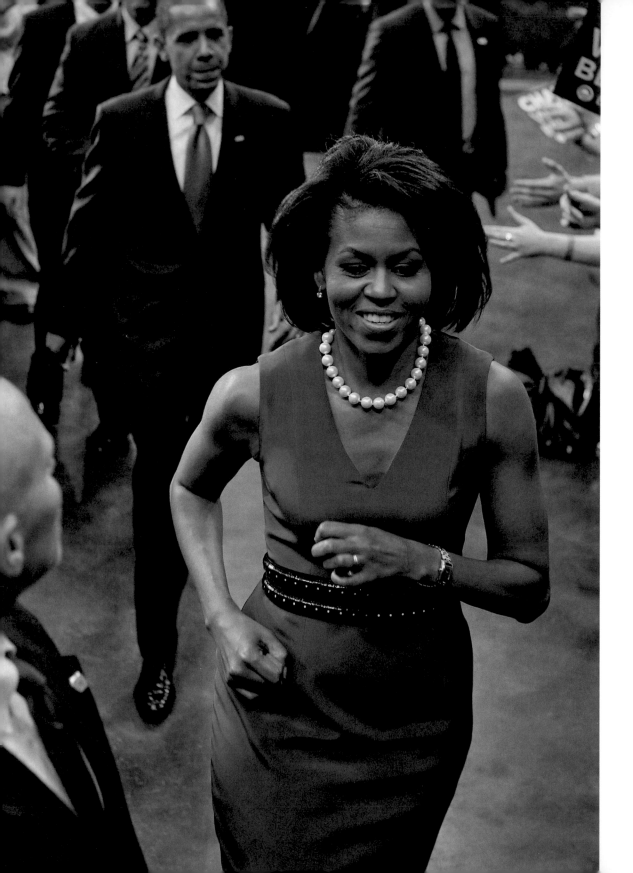

The successful route to a strong, healthy, and well-defined body is different for each of us, but critical for all of us. Obama is unabashedly honest about herself and has even gone on record noting in a recent interview with *Women's Health:* "I have to exercise and eat in a balanced way. If I start ignoring both, I will put on weight." Fitness pro and creator of such inspirational exercise videos as *Sweating in the Spirit* and *Body Gospel,* Donna Richardson Joyner was recently appointed to the Presidential Council on Fitness, Sports, and Nutrition under President Obama. She believes there has to be a paradigm shift. "Your thoughts govern your actions, so if you're going to change, you have to want to change more than you want to stay the same," she concludes. For certain, determination is the key to mastering your health and wellness. Being First Lady doesn't make it any easier for Michelle Obama to get up at 4:30 a.m. to work out than it does for any of us. But she does with informed determination. Michelle gives herself to Michelle—a free stretch of time that she sets aside to do for self before she gives herself to the world.

MIKKI-ISMS

Repeat after me:
Drop the excuses —
pick up the weights.

Working out in the morning works for her and is a smart strategy for any busy woman, plus it energizes you and allows you to hit the ground running. When it comes to nutrition, Mrs. O's good health efforts could easily be sabotaged by the number of events on her calendar. Imagine what life would be like if you accepted invitations to multiple social events close to 365 days a year! We lament over the fast five pounds we gain between Thanksgiving and New Year's and, that's just a matter of weeks. Try holding it down all year! The First Lady, who believes each of us has an individual responsibility to look after ourselves and our families by making better choices, practices what she preaches. Obama's diet is essentially about achieving a balance and including a lot of fruits and vegetables. It also includes healthy soups and lots of salads. She's not orthodox in her approach, though, as she allows for having a treat such as a plate of French fries occasionally, including the sweet potato fries the White House chefs turn out. The First Lady believes that occasional treats are not only healthy, but also recommended. The campaign is also about portion control, something that she and health experts believe has gotten out of control. Most of us underestimate the amount of food we eat and overestimate what the recommended portion sizes in a meal should be.

The First Lady also uses a short cleansing diet, which includes only vegetables to detox her body. According to the White House, the First Lady's cleanse involves eating as many fruits and vegetables as possible and cutting out fats, oil, dairy, meat, caffeine, sugar, and starch for a short period of time. This she does as way to "clean out her palate," as she's said, and to keep her sugar cravings in check. Looking at our empowered sister, one can see it not only takes discipline but also a different perspective on eating altogether. We in the United States are bombarded with television commercials about food and attached to the idea of food as reward, central to socializing and comfort. It's no wonder there's so much information coming forth about emotional eating. But if we're going to

MIKKI-ISMS

Change your definition of "reward" — it's not a chocolate bar or a latte — it's reaching a milestone. A reward is a relaxing bath at the end of the day, in other words, something that builds you up and does not break down your body, mind, and spirit with guilt and undo challenges.

master the art of eating well, then we must place our focus on the nutritional and healing value of food and drink to reset our thinking about what's acceptable and what's not.

Dr. Rovenia M. Brock, a.k.a. "Dr. Ro," an award-winning health journalist, television personality, and nutrition coach, waxes long and hard on our need to change and begin incorporating lots of colorful vegetables into our diet. "We need to get more color in our diet because the pigments have chemical compounds, phytochemicals and antioxidants, in them that go a long way to protect us from the diseases that disproportionately affect us." Ro is also big on organic produce, particularly those fruits, such as apples, whose skin contains a soluble fiber called pectin that can protect against heart disease by making your arteries more supple. The issue of whether a food is organic is more important in some cases than others, especially when you're eating the skins of produce. "I don't care if the oranges you consume aren't organic, because you're going to peel the skin. The problem is the pesticides found in the skins of fruits and vegetables that have a tendency to disrupt your endocrine function which can cause weight gain."

I know firsthand the challenges of eating healthy. I used to be in bondage to my taste buds and addicted to the pleasure of mindless eating to relieve stress. But when you learn better, you do better. I've come to know my triggers—sweets, cookies, cakes, and breads (all represent sugar cravings) and those times when I'm on overload, taking on more than I should. I've also studied my family's history, and I know that heart disease, high blood pressure, and strokes run in my family—on both sides. Armed with that awareness, I can't afford to eat carelessly. Ignorance is not bliss. In reality, ignorance is a dangerous form of kidding one's self. And just like a First Lady, we all need support. Losing sight of privately held goals is easy to do otherwise. In fact, we all need what I call a "temple management" team. That is a handpicked group of experts to keep you operating at your best, within and without. My temple management team includes my medical doctor, iridologist (a health practitioner who uses the patterns of your eye's iris to reveal the condition of your body), nutritionist, and personal trainer. They teach me which foods to eat and avoid and how to be in tune with my body to recognize symptoms such as bloating, sluggishness, inflammation, irritability, and unwanted pounds that signal problems. That means I try to avoid all forms of sugar, because

MIKKI-ISMS

*Don't kid yourself: when it comes to **mastering good health**, it helps to be a little **vain**.*

it always takes more than it gives. I also avoid salt, as there's far too much salt in the American diet as it is just by the mere fact that it's added to *everything*. I don't need to add more. My healthy practices include the use of herbs, garlic, and the occasional salt substitute when cooking for my family. I get my share of protein from fish, beans, egg whites, and occasionally skinless chicken. I make sure that my diet is rich in fruits, vegetables, healthy grains, nuts, and seeds. My daily supplements and lots of water are important to my regime as well. And I'm a big proponent of food combining. I only eat protein with veggies or veggies with carbohydrates, never all three together. This keeps my enzymes working at an optimal level. Experts like Dr. Ro feel strongly about proper food combinations.

We also need to tighten up our eating habits in terms of timing. Spend any amount of time talking to Ro, and she'll convince you that you must consume the bulk of your calories early in the day. According to Ro, cortisol levels begin to peak between 3:00 and 6:00 in the afternoon. She explains that "those stress hormones, which are cortisols, will cause you to have cravings for high-fat, high-sugar foods, so you start wondering why you're craving potato chips, ice cream, and all that kind of stuff."

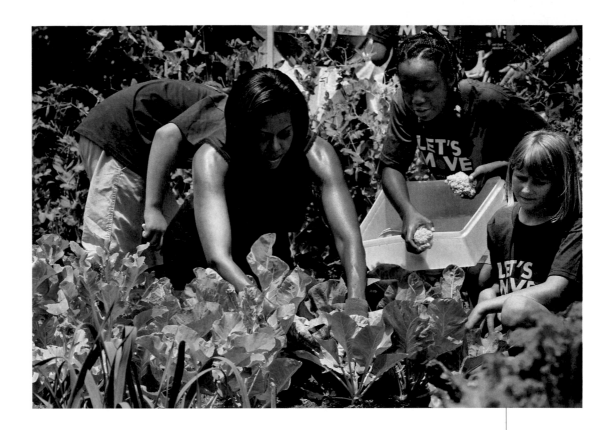

She adds, "If you do consume those foods, you will start to put on weight in the belly region." And as Manhattan iridologist Sally Kravich reminds us, "Belly fat is linked to heart disease and Type 2 diabetes." I'm learning the value of consuming more protein, particularly later in the day and definitely at dinner. For me that means having a boiled egg with my veggie juice and lean protein with a leafy green at dinner rather than the granola and raisins or oatmeal cookies that I love!

A healthy lifestyle is a pursuit for me, and the more I learn, the more I want to know. A few years ago, I was determined to boost my energy level without stimulants such as coffee and energy drinks. While interviewing various experts, I learned about the value of raw juicing and that was one of those moves that forever changed my life and the quality of my health. I visited the Martha's Vineyard Holistic Retreat for a reawakening and since that time, nothing else has been the same. According to Dr. Roni DeLuz, naturopathic doctor, founder of Martha's Vineyard Holistic Retreat, and author of the *New York Times* bestseller *21 Pounds in 21 Days: The Martha's Vineyard Diet Detox*, vegetables were put on earth as a cleansing food. "Vegetables de-inflate us," she says citing one of the benefits of juicing raw veggies. And in this day and age when eating nine servings of fruits and vegetables is the recommended daily requirement, juicing can make achieving that easier, "while gaining maximum nutrition and vital nutrients in small doses." Today, juicing is an essential part of my life—one that sees me rising early to juice a variety of veggies, particularly Eden-like greens of collards, kale, spinach, and broccoli—all rich in vitamins and nutrients. To these I add a variety of extras like apples, lemon, yellow and red beets, parsley, cilantro, cucumber (a natural diuretic), ginger, carrots, and whatever else I know is going to polish my temple from the inside out. When on the go, I add protein shakes that are a mix of protein powder, coconut water, and rice milk. I don't do cow's milk, since regardless of what anyone says, I know the cow's milk is for her calf—not me. I find it strange that humans are the only mammals that consume the milk of other mammals. When you think about it, the calf has to stand on its legs within hours of its birth. That's not our truth—go figure. When traveling, I don't do fast food. Instead I do my homework, researching health food markets and juice bars in advance of my travels so my healthy habits are also along for the ride. I don't drink alcohol at all, so fortunately I don't have to figure that into my equation. Again, it's all about determination and a focused mind-set.

Commander in Chic

YOU BETTER WORK IT!

When it comes to exercise, one of the most meaningful first steps you can take is to find a form that you enjoy. Once you do, staying motivated will no longer be an issue. The benefits of exercise are well documented and experts are adding to the list with each new study. According to Beverly Hills–based personal trainer and author of *The Workout*, Gunnar Peterson, each of us should "train like you're younger than you are. Don't say well I'm fifty, I can't do this exercise that I did when I was forty," he adds.

Mrs. O is certainly doing her part to get us to move not only by following a diligent regimen, but by the testimony of a strong, well-toned body with energy to spare. I can't begin to tell you how inspired I am when I see those photo ops where she's working a hula hoop (a sure sign of strong abs!), skipping hopscotch (a sign of great balance), jumping rope, or catching a football during the NFL's Play 60 campaign. She really is demonstrating to us that we can be active in a healthy way. She knows full well that you can't burn the candle at both ends and function at a high level. Obama says she goes to bed early at night as she rises early to work out. She described herself as not a night person in an interview with Barbara Walters. The interview was an "aha moment" for me, reminding me of the connection between adequate sleep and reduced cortisol. Remember, this is the hormone that courses through our bodies when we're stressed or don't get enough sleep and is associated with cravings and belly fat.

Cornell McClellan, fitness consultant and Personal Trainer to the First Family, takes Mrs. O through an intense weight-training routine made up of compound movements that work multiple muscle groups. An average workout might include one set of 15 to 20 reps each of lunges,

MIKKI-ISMS

What's fabulous? Getting older— but not old.

WORD PERFECT

Mastering your health and wellness is about appraising your vessel from an informed perspective and exercising the smartest options that will move you from where you are to where you want to be. "You have to eat the right food, do the right amount and the right kinds of exercise, and have the right lifestyle behaviors—for example, not smoking, not consuming too much alcohol, avoiding the things that are harmful to your body," says Dr. Ian K. Smith. Clearly there's a nutritional aspect to wellness, a psychological aspect to wellness, and a physical aspect to wellness. "And if you want to achieve optimal wellness, then you have to try to be at your best in all of those categories," Smith concludes. So you have to make the investment. Here's the *word* on what's key:

- Know your health stats and be clear about your objectives.

- Don't operate in isolation: Establish a temple management team of those essential professionals to support your health and wellness.

- Don't be afraid of consistent checkups. Be the *partner* in your health.

- Keep to a healthy weight—ask your team what that figure is based on your height and inner health.

- Be determined to eat for your health by consuming lots of organic fruits, vegetables, beans, and whole grains. Eat organic chicken, turkey, and lean meats. Eat two to three servings of low-mercury fish (wild salmon, tilapia, or catfish) per week.

- Eliminate organ meats, unhealthy fats, and packaged or processed foods.

- Limit your sodium intake!

- Be a mindful eater: be aware of why you're eating, what you're eating, and how much. Watch your food portions and slow your pace, making sure to chew food slowly and thoroughly.

- Consume small meals as opposed to the old-school practice of "three meals a day." This is the best way to burn fat, increase energy, and stave off cravings for snacks and sweets.

- Make it a point to exercise four to six times a week.

- Take supplements that are targeted to meet your needs as determined by a health care professional.

- Broil, grill, and bake foods; don't fry.

- Reduce stress—through exercise, deep breathing techniques, meditation.

- If you smoke, *stop*. Smoking is one of the major risk factors associated with heart attack, cancer, and stroke.

- Don't skimp on sleep, since doing so impacts your immune system, stimulates cravings, and is linked to increased belly fat, which is directly linked to heart disease.

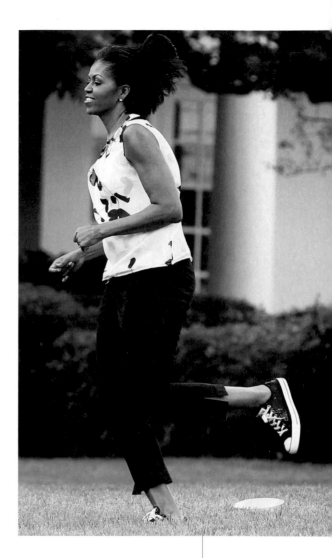

- Tend your emotional health by taking consistent, restorative "time for self."

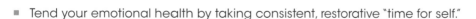

bench presses, hip raises, and rows—with short bouts of intense cardio mixed in. For an even greater total-body challenge, the workouts also feature rope-jumping, kickboxing, and body-weight calisthenics, all done at a heart- and lung-busting pace that skyrockets fitness levels and burns tons of calories.

Being fit and healthy requires a daily practice that supports your goals. Exercise impacts body weight, builds lean muscle, promotes strong bones and joint development, and strengthens our immune system, making it more able to fight off illness and disease. And when combined with a healthy diet, it can help prevent many chronic diseases including heart disease, cancer, and strokes. Finally, exercise also releases endorphins, those "feel good" molecules that lift our spirits and reduce stress.

Like many of us, I used to think I didn't have time to exercise. What I learned was that neglecting to do so was a real form of deprivation to both my mental and physical health, let alone my waistline. Now exercise is something that I look forward to with the passion of a child heading out to play. My regimen is to work out for thirty to sixty minutes twice a week with my personal trainer, focusing on strength, muscle tone, and flexibility. During our sessions, we box, lift weights, do TRX (a form of suspension training), kinesis, and more. In addition, three to five days a week I'm engaged in some type of hourlong cardio session that puts calories through the fire—whether a spin class, kickboxing, boot camp, or hitting the treadmill or the track for miles. The child in me also loves the Rebounder, which is a great form of cardio. As my awareness of the benefits of stretching and flexibility exercises increases, I'm including Pilates and yoga in my regime. Most of all, I'm having fun in the process, while getting tight, strong, and energized. The fact that I can boldly wear the looks I choose and that my arms don't keep waving at someone once I've stopped is pretty sweet, too.

Commander in Chic

As women shaping the world, we must do so by example. In truth, we are nurturers by nature, it's in our DNA. What we have to become comfortable with—and well informed about—is redirecting the care we give so well to others back to ourselves. Holistic health counselor, fitness and nutrition powerhouse Latham Thomas reminds us to prioritize the value of self-care. "When you take care of yourself first and foremost," she says, "you can be of amazing service to others." When we don't shift our thinking and actions accordingly, we suffer. It's as Sally Kravich says, "We can't keep giving from an empty well and not replenish ourselves." It's about making that all-important time for self—it's getting used to seeing your name on your schedule, and if that's what it takes to make it happen, pen yourself in. Latham encourages us all to "find the practices—tennis, dance classes, Pilates, running—that resonate with you and do those things each day, or at least a couple of times a week." We all stand to benefit by creating a new legacy: one that recognizes the value of self-nurturing.

While reaching our goals and overcoming what may at times seem like insurmountable challenges, we ultimately hold the "owner's manual" to our bodies and must choose to define them in ways that will allow them to serve us well in the journey. Look challenges in the face and deal with them—whether it's the illnesses that run in your family or the dead zones of the supermarkets—the tempting aisles of packaged and processed foods—or at the fast-food restaurants at every corner we turn. As personal trainer Gunnar Peterson is often fond of reminding, "Your body wasn't designed to process processed foods." So just say no.

We need more personal accountability. As Joyner puts it, "I want people to be faithfully fit and fabulous." The Bible says, "Faith without works is dead." No one of us is above the need to be disciplined about our health maintenance, including our icons like Beyoncé and Mary J. Blige.

"They don't have the 'Get out of being fat' card," says Kacy Duke, author of *The Show It Love Workout*. "They have lives and woes and things that they are going through, but they have to chin it up, and they have to get out there and do what they have to do," she concludes. So do we.

All in all, the critical work each of us must do is own our actions as it pertains to our health and wellness. Like one who is empowered, we should exercise our options and commit to working out for our health's sake on a daily basis once we receive a clear approval from our medical practitioner. Establishing concrete goals, lowering and maintaining a healthy weight by eating lean and becoming physically active all can help close the gap between where you are and where you need be. As Mrs. O told the children at Newark, New Jersey's, Maple Avenue School: "You got to be healthy if you're going to change the world, right?"

WORK IT OUT: YOUR GUIDE TO EXERCISING YOUR BEST AT ANY AGE

During my first cover shoot with the Obama family, then-Senator Obama stopped to admire Michelle while she was being photographed. I glanced over at him as he stood on the porch with his arms folded. He bore the biggest smile and a gleam in his eyes. That told a story of love and admiration that I'll never forget. Our future president was like a teenager all over again, smitten by his sweetheart as he stood there saying, "Isn't she cute!" Watching her blush at his reaction while trying to stay focused on being photographed was just priceless. She posed for the camera in a purple sheath, looking trim, toned, and baring those fabulous arms. Mrs. O was a picture of complete confidence. Part of that sense of assurance comes from investing in oneself and then playing it forward. Obama bares her arms like a twenty-something because they are just as tight. She can step out in a pair of shorts without thinking twice because every inch of her long legs is well toned. And yes, she can wear a sheath or a body-glove of a dress with that enviable figure because she works at maintaining it, and she's been at it for a long time. Her focused efforts and great discipline show. Mrs. O is living proof that age is just a number. "You have to become the architect of your own body," celebrity fitness pro Kacy Duke reminds us. In so doing, know that you can train yourself to work out at any hour, but if you're a morning person—use it. If you "come to life" after hours—go for it, just make sure you don't work out too close to bedtime, as it's not the time to be energized! However, if you're just beginning what should be a lifelong commitment to taking care of yourself, here's a guide from the pros to exercising your best options at any age.

Your Twenties

Your metabolism is revved up and you're strong. This doesn't mean that you can get away with eating unhealthy and not exercising. "The reality is once you hit twenty-two, the metabolism slows down," says Duke.

Your RX. Get moving with cardio five times a week. Try African dance classes, Zumba, belly dancing, Vinyasa, rope-jumping, running, spinning—make it fun. Cardio revs up your metabolism, burns calories, and strengthens your heart and lungs. "You should also be engaged in strength-training exercises," says Joyner, to keep muscle and bone strong and prevent osteoporosis. Engage in some form of weight training three times a week whether using free weights, weight-bearing equipment, or suspension training, which uses your own body weight as resistance. (Note: Dance is also a weight-bearing exercise.)

Your Thirties

Your metabolism really starts to slow down and, according to Smith, muscle mass is reduced. Weight doesn't come off as easily as before. Part of the tendency to retain weight at this age is also due to gender-related anatomical and physiological differences or what Smith considers "the mechanics of life development," which includes hormonal changes and pregnancies.

Your RX. Getting and staying fit means exercising five times a week and doing cardiovascular exercise in particular to counteract the effects of aging. This is the time when you want to mix it up and keep your body guessing so it won't get used to a routine. Kickboxing classes, Gospel aerobics, boot camp sessions, and other types of high-intensity exercises sustained for the course of an hour will leave you craving more in no time. Weight training exercise is also crucial, and experts like Duke recommend body-sculpting classes and enlisting the support of a personal trainer so you can add variety and challenge to your workout two to three times a week on the same day as your cardiovascular workouts or on the day in between. Building long, strong, and lean muscles is also important and Pilates, yoga, and Yogilates will give you essential strength, tone, and flexibility.

Your Forties

This is the decade of change and one Duke refers to as "heavy-duty time," as your hormones begin to prepare for the "rites of passage," she says, of menopause. During the forties your metabolism is definitely slower, the pull of gravity is starting to show, and your bone density is decreasing. "And that just means that you got to do a little more—it's going to happen, and you know it and you feel it and your body signals it—so tell yourself, I just have to do more to maintain what I have," says Joyner.

Commander in Chic

Your RX. "If you're trying to lose weight, you've got to be doing some type of cardiovascular exercise at least four to six times a week, thirty to sixty minutes each day," says Joyner. Here, "variety is the spice of life," and the more you mix it up, especially with those classes that make you feel sexy and empowered like Tae Bo, Zumba, or belly dancing, the more you'll see progress and be motivated to adhere to the process. You will also want to increase your weight-bearing and strength-training sessions to three times a week. Ditto for stretching and flexibility exercises, which are paramount now. Flexibility training is often neglected because its benefits aren't quite as apparent, but the average female adult loses 40 percent of her flexibility between the ages of twenty and seventy so it's a worthwhile investment that truly pays off when it comes to your joints.

Your Fifties

Sisters who are in great shape are fond of saying "fifties are the new thirties." Certainly today's generation of savvy, actively engaged age fifty-plus beauties are a very different group than those of generations past. Despite the fact that you're going through menopause and seeing belly fat a little more due to your cortisol levels, your zest for life and the knowledge you bring to the table are enviable. Duke says women in their fifties should have this motto: "Keep your past as your teacher, the present as your creation, and the future as your inspiration!"

Your RX. Be passionate about working out now. After all, this is "arrival time" and you are your own brand and calling card! Mix up your workouts and "focus on strength training and stretching for flexibility twice a week," encourages Dr. Smith. Load your iPod and aim for cardio exercises four to six times a week, whether through riding a stationary bike or a power-walk through the park with other sister-friends, then flip it and take a step-aerobics or Rebounder class or an energetic aqua-aerobics session.

TAKING STOCK: HOW TO MAKE THAT ALL-IMPORTANT NUDE ASSESSMENT

Being confident in your body requires both honesty and appreciation. Don't take the approach where you first put on your bathing suit after a "long winter's nap" and feel defeated. Use this opportunity to examine yourself without judgment as a way of researching your needs. Assessing yourself in the nude can be the beginning of a journey to your best body—here's how to approach it:

- Get naked in a three-way mirror and get to know your body. If you have any insecurity about any areas, ask yourself why. Analyze what it would take to make improvements and become comfortable in your own skin. Accept the wondrous vessel you've been given by your Creator and set your intentions on nurturing your body right then and there.

- Recognize that you are more than a dress size or any other measurement that doesn't take into account your greatness in the eyes of God who made you in His image. Appraise your body from that perspective.

- Be thankful for clarity and start a new conversation with yourself that cancels the negative and embraces the positive. Support the mindset with real change through exercise, healthful eating, and spiritual practices that support your emotional well-being.

- Overcome insecurities about any body part. There's always a way to rule in the positive. If you have a sleeveless dress you love, but your arms are too soft—grab a shrug; if your great abs are concealed by a belly right now—work a tunic. In other words, keep it moving, Sis. Work well with what you have. Life is too short to take pause!

- Give your insecurities to charity! Clean out your closet and give away those clothes that don't fit properly to someone who could be enjoying them. Replace those pieces with clothing that makes you look great now and feel fabulous.

- Venture out of your comfort zone. If you always wear black, strike change with color. Work a monochromatic hue like navy or bordeaux, head to toe, or turn up the heat when you do wear black by adding a shock of color to play up your assets.

- Dress to celebrate *your* figure. If you've got great arms—work them in sleeveless sheaths, elegant tops, and fitted sleeves. Possess great legs? Work them in age-appropriate hemlines that shape or move coupled with conversation-worthy footwear. Whittled waistline? Make it count with fabulous belts, shaped jackets, and curve-conscious dresses.

- Finally, use that mirror for something other than calling attention to areas designated for improvement by penning notes of self-affirmation and place them there with an attitude of gratitude—a fabulous way to greet yourself in the buff each day.

MIKKI-ISMS

Stay ready for your close-up: get a three-way mirror and be informed.

LEANER, STRONGER, SEXIER: TIPS TO EXERCISING YOUR BEST ASSETS

Because her focused and effective workouts allow her to be a style liberal, the First Lady can bare her arms, skip hose, and cinch her waist on any given day of the week with an attention-getting belt. Such results are not achieved by isolated exercise, otherwise known as spot-toning. Doing 200 situps a day and no other form of exercise is not effective for optimum fitness. You cannot spot-reduce fat. What you can do, however, is turn up the heat on those body parts you deem your best assets as part of your *overall* workout regimen. Include cardio and resistance exercises, and a healthy eating plan to be fit and healthy. And remember, when strength training, allow for a day of rest in between such workouts.

Aerobic and Fitness Association of America Fitness Pro and personal trainer Pierre S. Docsol shares a few surefire moves to help you accentuate the fabulous.

Arms. Up the ante with bicep curls; here's how: Stand feet shoulder-width apart, holding a dumbbell in each of your hands, palms facing your body. Make sure your shoulders are down and relaxed and abs are tight. Turn your wrists so that your palms face forward. Bend elbow, then slowly raise the weights up to shoulder height. Slowly lower the arms and repeat; challenge yourself to do 3 sets of 12 to 15 reps using weights no fewer than 15 pounds.

Commander in Chic

Legs. Build killer legs with the sumo squat. Sit on the bench with a weight between your legs, and making sure your knees do not go over your toes. Stand up, then sit back down; make sure to keep your chest up as you do. Do 3 sets of 15 to 20 reps.

Waist/Abs. Assume the "power plank" position; here's how: Using a mat, lie facedown on the floor, then come up on your toes and forearms with your shoulders and elbows lined horizontally so your body forms a straight line from your head to your heels. Hold this pushup-like position, making sure your back isn't arched and your abs don't droop, for 45 seconds building to a minute. Repeat for 4 sets.

Derriere. Keep it firm with lunges; here's how: Stand straight with your feet hip-width apart; step about 4 feet backward with your right foot, creating a 90-degree angle, making sure the bent knee is directly over your ankle. Repeat for a full set of 12, then switch and repeat on the other side.

Back. Firm it pretty with the reverse fly. Sit on the edge of a bench, a 5-pound weight in each hand with your chest on your lap, and extend your arms up as if flying. Do 3 sets of 15 reps.

MIKKI-ISMS

Find your fighting spirit and work it out.

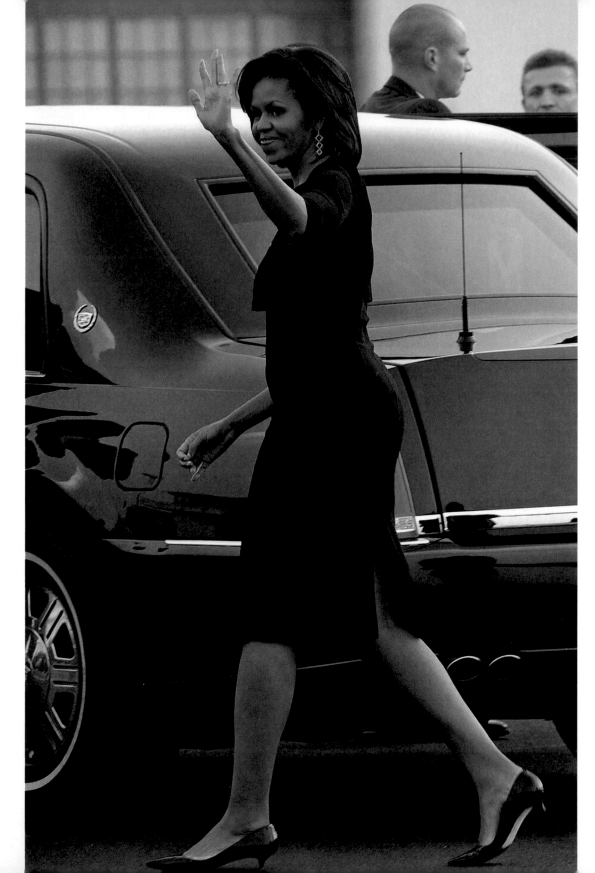

5

STYLE-TO-GO

There's something empowering about the reality-checked way in which Michelle Obama works fashion. From her courting of the best chic and inexpensive finds, to those big nights at "home" that see her *info-taining* people from all walks of life dressed by the most seasoned designers, she makes you want to rethink everything you ever knew about great style. No matter what she's wearing, there's always an inherent sense of effortless chic about the way she puts a look together and how she carries it. I simply can't imagine her at the end of any day being ready to collapse from any restricting, uncomfortable garment she had on. Like any well-dressed woman, she knows who she is and who she isn't, and she doesn't waver. This is why her wardrobe works wherever life takes her, whether to Paris, France, or Mexico City—and any other point on the globe, for that matter. Take your pick, and there's an Obama look worth your attention, no matter the climate, the occasion, or the hour. She always emerges from Air Force One looking picture perfect, because she wears clothing that is relevant to how she lives her life. It's really a form of the best style-to-go—smart, chic, wearable. Qualities like these have redefined glamour as we know it in the age of Michelle Obama, from one that was previously based on red-carpet sensibilities (and how many of us really have to worry about what to wear on the carpet?) to one that makes sense for our modern, purposeful lives. She is not loyal to one designer or even just a few. Her great looks can't be explained by an endless flow of cash. Unfortunately, we've all seen presidential wives who shot their wad in the wrong fashion direction! I'm just saying!

A LIFE IN STYLE

By Day

Editor's Picks:

A SMART DRESS | A MULTITASKING CARDI | A CHIC ENSEMBLE

The First Lady calls on her favorite staples for her workdays, no matter what's on her schedule. On the following pages, we see her bankable buys: a great dress, the cardi, and the trusted ensemble of a smart coat and matching sheath. They represent my picks and your takeaways as these pieces anchor a wardrobe and all allow one the kind of polished, pulled-together style essential in her day-to-day. Whether you're a young executive on the rise or a CEO, who doesn't need a smart, effortless dress that you can always count on? As we've seen again and again, a great cardi is a multitasker in that it can add sophistication to a look during the week and then become your best casual player on the weekend. An ensemble is a match made in heaven, in that the coat works over a great dress and on its own, whether over a chic pair of trousers or flared pants or a plethora of great skirts. The dress is magic solo or again can work with a great cardi or a smart jacket. You can also can change its character from minimalist and chic to soigné and sophisticated with a simple change of accessories.

This equation for modern dressing represents one that is smart, let alone quite simple. With pieces like these as your base, you can shop at all price points, mixing high and low, just like Mrs. O, and enjoy the experience. In truth, who has the time to obsess about what they're going to wear anymore? I know every time I've worked with the First Lady in preparation for a shoot, I have one conversation regarding the style directive for the look and her team pulls it, just like that! The same holds true for the range of celebs and corporate leaders I know and have had the pleasure of working with. Their closets are ordered and I can go in with my team and pull multiple looks without having to conduct a "shop"—and not because of what money affords them, but rather due to the clear sense each has of what works for them. In fact, one of my prominent sister-friends' closet is so tightly edited that moving her look from day to night is such a breeze that all she has to do is reach for a change of accessories and a lipstick!

Last, know that it's not about having a closet "full of clothes"—it's about having great options you can count on. Make it a point to know the pieces that work best on you and allow you to comfortably be your best at all times. I remember one frugal but fabulous sister told me years ago, "show me a woman with a closet full of clothes —i.e., trendy pieces —and I'll show you a woman who doesn't know how to dress."

MIKKI-ISMS

Choose your shopping partners wisely—personally I like "me, myself, and I." Other than that only a good, honest girlfriend will do.

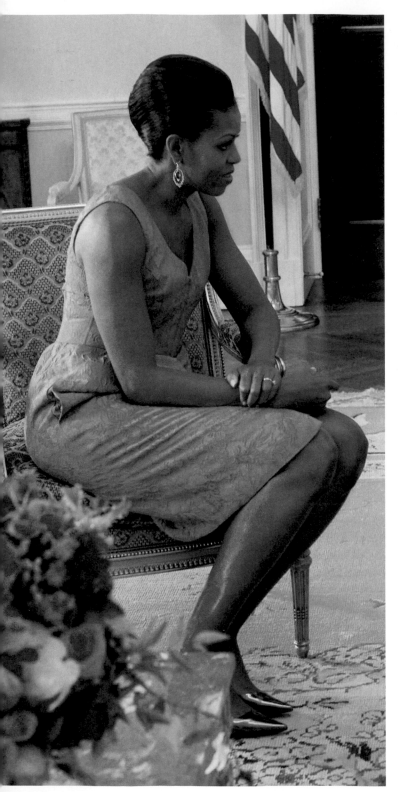

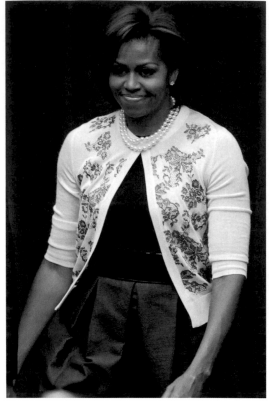

BY DAY *Easy, chic style is on everyone's "most wanted" list, and the First Lady nails it with star buys that simply work. Looks like this dress and matching coat represent a strong style message worn together or paired exquisitely with other separates. The embellished cardi, with its retro-esque sensibility is timeless yet directional, and can be reinterpreted by a change of accessories and any range of great basics. The sheath, an Obama signature, keeps her looking modern and polished. And, don't we, like Mrs. O, love a dress that's so simply fabulous it loses nothing when paired with a flat? Point worth noting!*

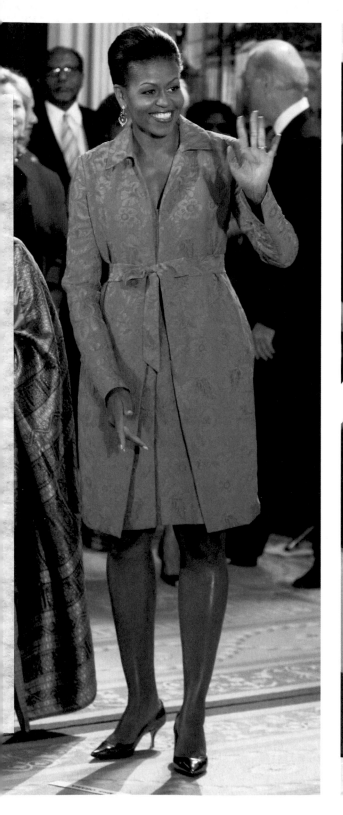
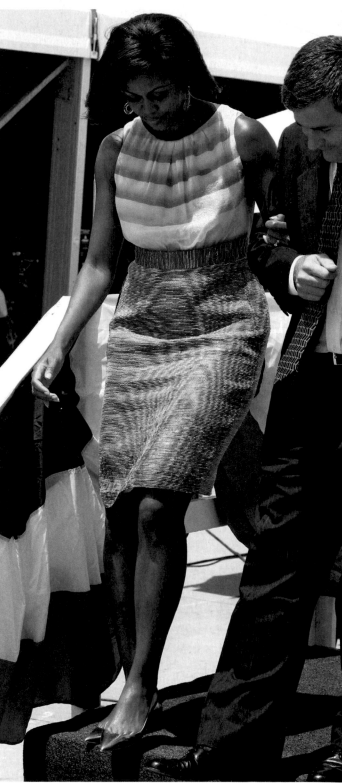

By Night

Editor's Picks:

A STUNNING COCKTAIL DRESS | SENSUOUS SEPARATES |
A TIMELESS GOWN

Whether she's stepping out at night or simply entertaining at the White House, Mrs. O masters a look that's always a standout. Though she often calls on her favorite LBDs, we see here that she also has a penchant for color, amazing neutrals, texture and shine, and silhos that range from structured to soft and floaty. The looks shown here represent my picks for after-hours perfection. I love the floral frock, as it's the way to light up the night again and again! The mood-thrilling hues and the ultra-feminine shaping are traffic-stopping! It's the kind of dress that makes one look forward to a great invitation. At the heart of its sensation is an impeccable fit, and that's the takeaway for any structured frock, no matter the price point, since it's the way to make sure it goes from "nice dress" to "amazing dress." If you're just starting to build your "black tie" wardrobe, separates can be a great investment. Take, for example, Obama's long, shimmery evening skirt cut on the bias and the sensuous silk blouse. The skirt can take on an array of tops—from beautiful blouses to tank silhos—even a sensuous cashmere sweater. Additions like this add mileage to your wardrobe and will keep you out of that "last-minute shopper" category, which usually results in overspending and hasty decision making. Then there's the timeless gown. Trends come and go, but unless you've got money to burn, go for a gown that's timeless. This refined, lipstick-red halter gown is in a class by itself—one thats endlessly fabulous.

For certain, evening dressing can present a challenge. Oftentimes, the invitations we receive leave us in the dark, so it's no wonder we underdress or overdress in our effort to be apropos. Here again, there's a confident way to make those social calls after sundown in a manner that's true to who you are and how you dress. First, know the silhouettes that flatter you and stick to them. When the occasion calls for cocktails, responding to this is as simple as wearing your little black dress or wearing an elegantly cut pantsuit to work and changing your accessories. When the invitation reads "festive attire," reach for a party-perfect piece, such as a great dress, in a colorful hue, or a soft skirt that moves and a beautiful blouse. If the invite calls for "black-tie," know that a gown isn't your only option, but richness must be a part of the equation. You can be just as formal in a stunning velvet, lace, beaded, or sequined dress, just take it easy when it comes to your accessories and remember that "less is more." Now if the occasion calls for "white-tie," then a floor length gown is your option.

Evening hours call for you to prep your look and your closet ahead of time. It's about keeping your after-dark pieces ready to go with great maintenance—from dry-cleaning services to shoe and handbag repairs. It's also about making those strategic buys that will allow you to show up ready for each and every occasion. For example, add the duster coat we talked about in chapter 1 to your evening collection in black taffeta, get that black cashmere cardi the next time you see one on sale, and be sure to secure a timeless stole. Speaking of stoles, do take a page from the Obama style aesthetic and wear it well. When bearing her arms, for nighttime occasions Mrs. O usually calls on a featherweight stole to accompany the look, but always lets it rest effortlessly. Finally, unless you're onstage or working a red carpet, do forego a train. It's so not worth it to have every Tom, Dick, and Harry, and Jane of course, constantly stepping on it!

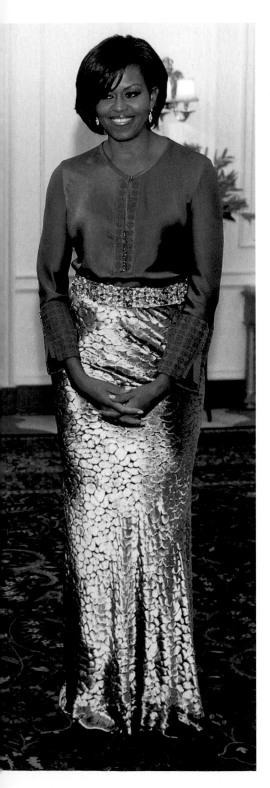

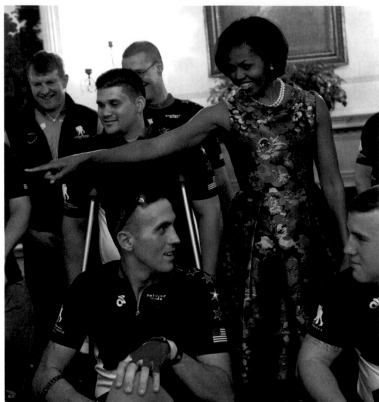

BY NIGHT *Mrs. O's life is full of "social calls." Yet she doesn't make the mistake of changing her style in an effort to pull out all the stops. Obama maintains her fashion mode as such, and always steps into the night with flawless aplomb. For receptions, she often chooses a great dress and equally great accessories—from a modern strand of pearls to a drop earring that peaks through her hair and completes the look, rather than taking over. At times, she'll pair the most elegant separates, as seen here, where a shimmery evening skirt is paired perfectly with a slip of a blouse and dazzling earrings. For state dinners and white-tie affairs, it's always about a timeless gown in an unforgettable hue or sensuous texture.*

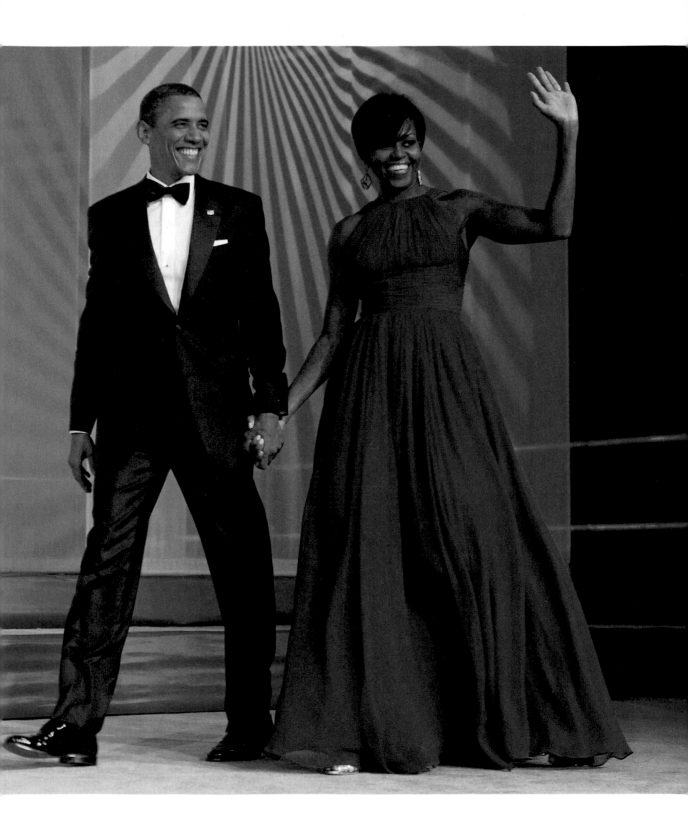

En Route

AN LBD | SNAPPY SEPARATES | EASY PIECES

Like many of us, Michelle is on the move as a wife and a mother, but she's also a woman who, just like any busy sister, works in that essential down-time to renew and restore. No matter where she's headed, she's always dressed effortlessly smart and easy, even when she's traveling. The selections shown here are my "keep it chic and simple" Obama faves. Clearly, there are those times when she has to step off the plane ready to go. I love how she slipped into this little black knit dress—it's a no-brainer. Just pair it with the perfect kitten heels for style and comfort and a strand of pearls, and you're so there. Who hasn't had to go straight from the plane to a meeting? This is one way to do so and not lose your style card! The snappy blazer popped over a pencil skirt and a sweater are just smart and easy. I also like how she added a great leather waist cincher to take it to the next level. These are timeless pieces that we all own, and when it comes to extending your wardrobe, it's just a question of how you play them forward in terms of creativity that matters most. Then there are the jersey separates that are perfect for travel, weekends, and more. You can take one pair of leggings and an array of tops and accessories and work a look from sporty to glam if you desire.

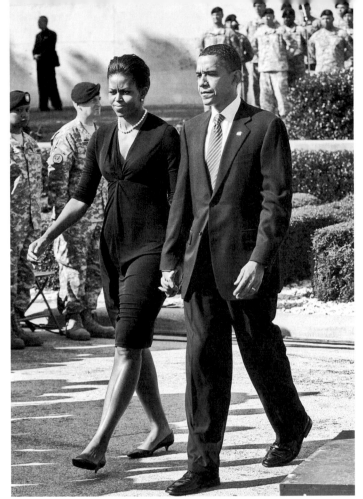

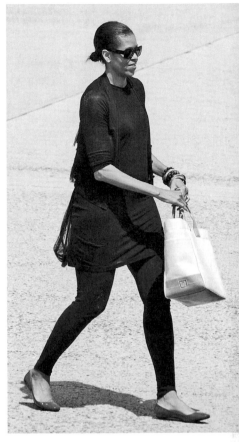

The First Lady proves you can look fab on or "off duty," with a well-thought-out wardrobe. This is not a new element to her fashion protocol—this has long been her plan of action. When traveling, comfort is important, but not at the expense of her style. Here Obama keeps it moving in an easy but elegant black knit dress. Her getaway style is fluid and effortless in breathable fabrics—from the fashionably fab tunic that moves to the cotton leggings. The black leather blazer is a smart, multitasker that works throughout her wardrobe and speaks to Michelle's underlying "fashion with a purpose" style ethic.

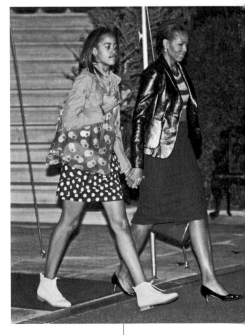

By Design

Find your fashion ease with Obama's consistent faves from A to Z.

Alexis Bittar, www.alexisbittar.com

Azzedine Alaïa, www.matchesfashion.com

Barbara Tfank, Barneys New York, www.Barneys.com

Carole Tanenbaum, www.caroletanenbaum.com

Carolee, www.carolee.com

Derek Lam, www.neimanmarcus.com

Diane von Furstenberg, www.dvf.com

Donna Karan, www.donnakaran.com

Erickson Beamon, www.ericksonbeamon.com

Isabel Toledo, select Nordstrom stores

Jason Wu, www.bergdorfgoodman.com

J.Crew, www.jcrew.com

Jimmy Choo, www.jimmychoo.com

Kevan Hall, www.kevanhalldesigns.com

L'Wren Scott, www.Barneys.com, Barneys New York in Beverly Hills,
    Barneys New York, NYC

Lanvin, Bergdorf Goodman, NYC; Lanvin Boutiques NYC
    and Los Angeles

Maria Pinto, Saks Fifth Avenue stores

Michael Kors, www.michaelkors.com

Moschino, www.moschinoboutique.com

Moschino Cheap and Chic, www.moschinoboutique.com

Narciso Rodriguez, www.bergdorfgoodman.com

Commander in Chic

Nina Ricci, Barneys New York stores, Bergdorf Goodman,
   Neiman Marcus

Peter Som, www.petersom.com

Ports 1961, www.ports1961.com

Prabal Gurung, Bergdorf Goodman, NYC,
   www.bergdorfgoodman.com

Rachel Roy, www.rachelroy.com

Thakoon, Bergdorf Goodman, NYC

Tom Binns, www.tombinnsdesign.com

Tracy Reese, www.tracyreese.com

Destination Style

The "in" spots that place Mrs. O's designers of choice at your fingertips:

Bergdorf Goodman, www.bergdorfgoodman.com

Bloomingdale's, www.bloomingdales.com

Charm & Chain, www.charmandchain.com

ikram, www.ikram.com

Lord & Taylor, www.lordandtaylor.com

Neiman Marcus, www.neimanmarcus.com

Nordstrom, http://shop.nordstrom.com

The Outnet, www.theoutnet.com

Saks Fifth Avenue, www.saksfifthavenue.com

shopbop.com, www.shopbop.com

The Bliss List

Looking for the chicest fashion finds at a low price? Here are the destinations where you can find fabulous sole mates, smart bags, and guilty pleasures that'll help you work a look like the first lady of style that you are and keep you coming back for more.

Ann Taylor, www.anntaylor.com

Anthropologie, www.anthropologie.com

ASOS, http://us.asos.com

Beyond the Rack, www.beyondtherack.com

Bluefly, www.bluefly.com

Boscov's, www.boscovs.com

Burlington Coat Factory, www.burlingtoncoatfactory.com

Century 21, www.c21stores.com

Daffy's, www.daffys.com

Designer Apparel, www.designerapparel.com

Dillard's, www.dillards.com

DKNY, www.dkny.com

Dolce Vita, www.shopdolcevita.com

DSW, www.dsw.com

Edwin Pearl, www.edwinpearl.com

Elder-Beerman, www.elder-beerman.com

Filene's Basement, www.filenesbasement.com

Gilt Groupe, www.gilt.com (Members only—but membership is free)

Halls Kansas City, www.halls.com

HauteLook, www.hautelook.com

H&M, www.hm.com

HSN, www.hsn.com

J.Crew, www.jcrew.com

Keds, www.keds.com

Kohl's, www.kohls.com

Loehmann's, www.loehmanns.com

Macy's, www.macys.com

Marshalls, www.marshallsonline.com

Max & Chloe, www.maxandchloe.com

Neiman Marcus Last Call, www.lastcall.com

Nine West, www.ninewest.com

Nordstrom Rack, www.shop.nordstrom.com/c/nordstrom-rack

OneStopPlus.com, www.onestopplus.com

OnlineShoes.com, www.onlineshoes.com

Payless, www.payless.com

QVC, www.qvc.com

Saks Fifth Avenue Off 5th, www.off5th.com

ShoptheLook.com, www.shopthelook.net

Stein Mart, www.steinmart.com

Syms, www.syms.com

Talbots, www.talbots.com

Target, www.target.com

T.J. Maxx, www.tjmaxx.com

Topshop, www.topshop.com

White House Black Market, www.whitehouseblackmarket.com

Zappos.com, www.zappos.com

Zara, www.zara.com

SHOP TALK

What constitutes smart shopping? Thinking like a style maven with go-to salespersons, a savvy list, strategic spending, a great eye for high and low finds and more! Here's how to score:

Take stock. Evaluate your wardrobe and have a clear idea of what you need before you shop. Don't purchase an entire new wardrobe each season but rather add specific pieces to build or refresh your wardrobe. Fill or replenish the essential basics you already own. Strategize and make a shopping list. Buy your investment pieces first, then the basic wardrobe fillers.

Know when to shop. Be there when the doors open, as you'll have the sales staff or your favorite salesperson all to yourself. Be aware of merchandise deliveries so you don't miss out. In general, spring fashion begins arriving in store in February and is in full throttle by March. Come June, as you're beginning to think about outdoor parties and fashion sales, early fall picks begin appearing. By August, fall is in and close on its heels are the most glittering holiday finds. Plan accordingly. For example, if you're in need of a great black "forever" clutch, know that between October and November the stores are on "overload" with items in the accessory and evening departments. So that's the time to buy. Ditto for that LBD you might want to add to your wardrobe. Know about sales *ahead* of time so you can take full advantage of them. Be on file at stores so you get the mailers in advance, but also know about the coupons and special discounts where they apply. Watch the papers so you'll have information on destinations you might not normally visit. Cultivate relationships with salespersons who will place your info on file for email alerts regarding sales and what's new in store.

Commander in Chic

Get VIP service. I schedule time with the various salespersons at the places I shop and as a result, the ladies always have a fitting room ready and waiting with the types of pieces they know I'll love and am looking for. This will save you time and money—from department stores and specialty boutiques to chain stores and outlet shops as well as those "vintage havens."

Keep your credit card on file. I'm a big believer in the practice of "charge and send," as it helps me avoid waiting in line, something I just haven't mastered yet! It's a good practice for those stores you trust and where you have a great salesperson at the ready.

ON THE ROAD—IN STYLE!

Can you imagine having to travel like the president's wife and not have someone to select and pack your wardrobe? Sounds overwhelming, right? Well, trust me, you may not have to travel like the First Lady, but whether you hit the road occasionally or routinely, you should be traveling in style, without effort, and with the kind of ease that a strategic packing formula ensures. Begin with an organized closet, no matter whether you have a walk-in or "a keep it simple space with two shelves at the top for storage," like me. My wardrobe and those of many of the high-profile women whose homes I frequent for imaging direction are set with a style-to-go approach in that everything is accessible. The clothing is hung in color categories, and all shoe boxes are labeled with a snapshot of the shoe on the front of the box or lined up on shoe shelves at-a-glance. The jeans are folded at the top, and handbags line the upper shelves. Now I do confess that I have a bag and shoe fetish, so all my "must-haves" that don't fit are accommodated in a lovely guest room.

So your first order of business is a well-organized closet, as this will allow you to pack at a moment's notice without getting flustered. What also helps is knowing what looks work well together and recording them so you don't have to think about it. For my clients, I organize their lives by establishing a "look book" that simplifies this task. For you, it's a matter of pulling out your camera or phone, snapping a shot of the look and accessories on your bed or on yourself with a smile, and recording it on your computer and, voilà, when you're ready to pack, you'll have an instant reference for what works. (I travel so much that I have standing packing lists on my computer for all of the cities and climates I frequent, so I'm halfway there whenever it's time to travel. This extra step also ensures I don't forget anything—from skin care to anything else I deem essential.)

The next step is putting it all together in a way that ensures you don't pack a million and one isolated looks and so many bags that your trip will cost you a fortune in luggage fees before you reach your destination. My friend Pamela Macklin says, "You're going away from home, not running away from home!" So think smart and think chic by choosing pieces that work well together and allow you to create a wardrobe of great looks from a minimal number of items. Then let accessories be the workhorses, allowing you to change your looks for different occasions and from day to night with ease. Here are some packing pointers to assist you in hitting the road in style:

Have a game plan. Check your "look book" for those outfits that you deem fabulous and appropriate for your destination and activities.

Review, review, review. Lay your looks out on the bed and see what you can edit—e.g., shoes that can be worn with various outfits, accessories that can work day to night, handbags that can multitask, etc.

Commander in Chic

Pack in neat, separate sections. Line folded items with acid-free tissue paper; shine leather shoes or brush suedes in advance, stuff with tissue-paper and store in shoe bags. Place lingerie and hosiery/socks in a lingerie bag. If you travel with a garment bag or a rollaway that's large enough to accommodate hanging garments, cover all items in plastic dry cleaner bags (on the hanger) and store in your luggage so that when you arrive, hanging them up is quick and easy. Store accessories in a jewelry pouch to make sure they aren't damaged in transit.

Looking good. Decant skin care into plastic, travel-size containers so you don't sacrifice your beauty routine just because you're away from home. I place hairbrushes and combs in large freezer bags to ensure they're well protected and place them into the corners of my luggage. Ditto for my travel steamer. You never know what you're going to find as an excuse for a good iron when you arrive at your hotel. Besides, ironing takes a toll on clothing, while steaming is such a kinder, gentler way to remove wrinkles and it will guarantee your pieces aren't scorched. Finally, pack a well-edited makeup bag in your carry-on, along with any other essentials, including thick socks (it's always cold on airplanes), travel blanket, and anything else you require for your comfort. Organize your in-flight outfit. I'm all about a casual-luxe approach so in winter, I love a great cashmere tunic and pants or jersey leggings, ballet flats, and a silk scarf to keep my do in check. In summer, I switch to cotton jersey cardis, a chic tunic, my CJ Joy legging jeans, and again ballet flats. I say make the most of your journeys by traveling stylishly. I've also found that looking polished and pulled together influences the kind of service I receive while traveling. You'll find that everyone—cabbies, airport personnel, bellmen, wait staff, etc.—will be promptly "at your service" when you travel in style.

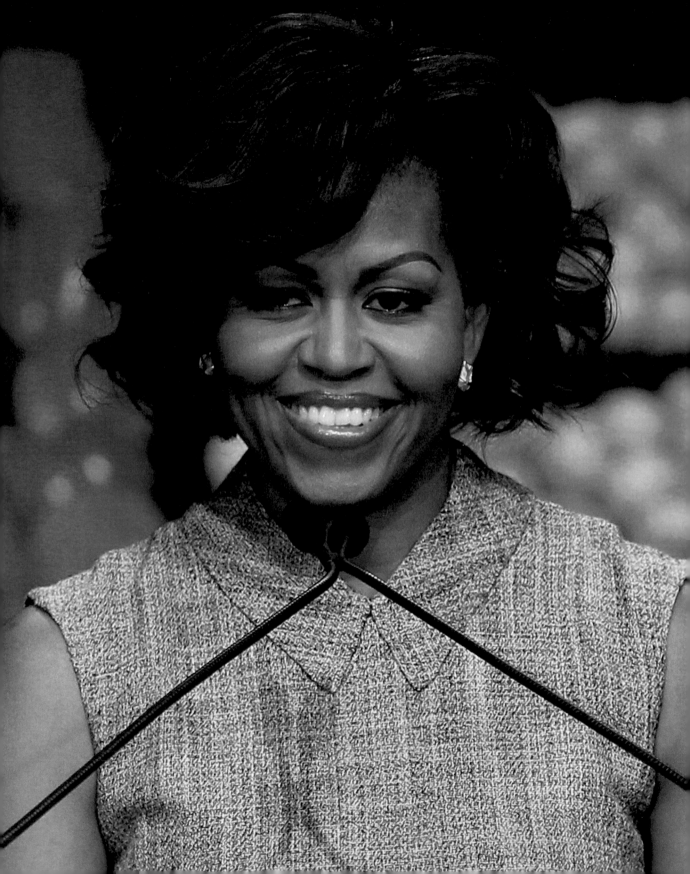

6

MAKE THE CUT!

When it comes to beauty, women in-the-know possess a clear knack for combining the timeless and the contemporary to create the most ultra-smart looks. Obama is no exception. Take, for example, her savvy, all-American bob: its workable length allows her the versatility necessary for her every desire. This ever-perfect cut works for her much like a little black dress in that it goes from day to night. She can swing it, softly set or pulled back into a retro-chic French roll or other great updos, and never fail to look polished and apropos. For the large percentage of us who have relaxed hair, a great cut and exceptional support products are key to maintaining a polished and healthy look. Partnering with a professional is also paramount to staying on point. Prior to stepping into the White House, Obama had a standing two-hour salon appointment every week at Chicago's Van Cleef Hair Studio. Likewise, your best-hair practices should include a customized care regimen, even if you're the one working it in between salon visits.

On a most basic level, a wise regimen of weekly shampooing and conditioning, trims every four to six weeks, and precise styling aids and tools should form the basis of your regime. And though Mrs. O's modern-day bob looks like an easy mane-stay, "Not so," says SoftSheen-Carson Artistic style director and celebrity hairstylist Johnny Wright. "It is the hardest cut to keep cut," he exclaims. Wright should know; he's not only in demand as stylist to the likes of Lauren London, LisaRaye McCoy, and Vivica A. Fox, but is also hairstylist to Michelle Obama. When asked "What's the secret to keeping a bob fresh, full, and glossy?" Johnny says, "It begins at the bowl with good shampoos and conditioners. From there it's about having the proper cut for volume." One trick of the trade he relies on is layering: "I often create layers in the crown to eliminate the weight because if the hair is too heavy or just cut as a straight A-line blunt cut, you're not going to be able to get the volume you want," he concludes. In watching Obama's very chic bob, you can't help but notice how it moves and look twice at its glossy finish, which shows off its precise layering throughout. Color techniques also play a role in terms of volume in that they give the illusion of thicker hair. Oftentimes when I'm in the studio creating various looks for the covers of *Essence*, our stylists will add highlights or lowlights through precolored or preselected extensions—which is another trick of the trade for such—as again, color lends dimension and the illusion of fullness. When you couple this with human-hair extensions, you also protect your hair from the perils of double processing.

Keeping a sharp crop beautiful and healthy also depends on discerning style practices. Without question, our hair is the most fragile on earth due to its natural curl pattern. When it is chemically processed, it becomes even more delicate and susceptible to breakage. This means that we have to choose the styling aids and practices that nurture our hair every step of the way. In truth, your styling aids and tools should be directed by your hair care professional. Shopping looks and labels is far too risky without knowing your hair type and its current condition—simply put, that is, what your hair can and *cannot* take. On any given day, we sisters have anywhere from three to four styling aids in our hair to polish and perfect our look, so it's essential that these products have synergy, that they don't weigh down our strands, or cause any adverse effects. Having a coterie of styling aids that you can trust is most important.

The same thinking applies to the maintenance and styling tools. They should be handpicked and used with a keen awareness as well. We know that repeated heat styling is dehydrating and over time breaks down the keratin of the hair. This translates to breakage, split ends, and lackluster locks, so when it comes to heat appliances, moderation is key. Keep temps moderate on flat irons; according to Wright, you shouldn't go higher than 350 degrees. Simple steps like not blow-drying your hair while it's dripping wet (blot it dry first with a microfiber hair towel) or opting for a roller set and incorporating the use of a hooded dryer can make a big difference as well. In addition, Wright recommends wrapping the hair at night to give it mold, instead of relying on the daily use of irons. An array of great style options that can be done quickly and without the use of heat is the best practice. As with Mrs. O, your cut should offer you the kind of flexibility that allows you to rock an array of looks as well as textures without taxing the health of your hair. Remember, your hair should reflect your style for every occasion and be well thought out. Your style strategy should be based on your hair type, condition, and lifestyle, including the amount of time you have to spend on your hair, whether you work out, and how much you travel. Which is why again, this approach should be determined by you and your stylist.

All in all, the freshest-looking hair is healthy, strategically maintained, and worn with confidence. There's simply nothing more alluring than a woman who knows what works for her and what doesn't, and, trust me, it shows up head to toe. One of my dearest friends calls it "staying in your lane." One look at Mrs. O says she's not only there, but moving full speed ahead.

GIVE ME 5: ONE BOB, FIVE GREAT TAKES

From full-on flirty to cool and curvaceous, Obama's above-the-collarbone cut is utterly fresh. Here's a look at several of the First Lady's style incarnations and what you need to know to make your own glam slam.

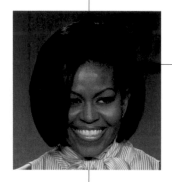

The Signature Staple: Classic, Full-Bodied, Curve Conscious

In salon: A symmetrical cut and a professional blow-dry using a round brush and a volumizing treat.

At home: Apply a volumizer and blow-dry hair using a round brush (only if you're adept at the technique). Otherwise, blow-dry hair upside-down using a comb attachment to create lift at the roots; bump hair (to coax lift at the roots and curve throughout) with a large-barrel curling iron or a flat iron whose plates have a slight curve to further add volume. Finish with a sheen spray.

Lush Layers, a Saucy, Lash-Grazing Bang, and High Shine Add a Sensuous Twist

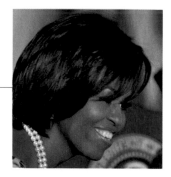

In salon: Soft, graduated layers are a must.

At-home: Wrap hair by night; in the a.m., set on large steam rollers, hand-style using a large-tooth comb to define layers. Finish with a sheen spray.

Asymmetrical Shaping Takes on Soft, Voluminous Curls

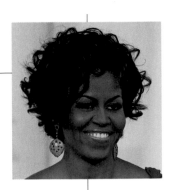

In salon: Figure 8 curls are created and hand-shaped to release and frame the face.

At home: Use a medium- to large-size curling iron or bevel hair with a small flat iron; finger-style into place with abandon!

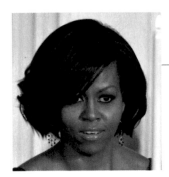

A Sweeping Asymmetrical Bang and a Soft, Hand-Combed Finish

In salon: A long sweep is flat-ironed into shape; tighter curls are set in place at the ends; the look is finished using a wide-tooth comb.

At-home: Wrap hair, set ends on steam rollers, comb into shape using a wide-tooth comb.

A Bouffant Crown and Unstudied Curls

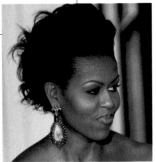

In salon: Root lifting is created at the crown for soft volume; hair is then swept off the face; figure 8 curls are created in back and pinned sporadically to form an elegant yet unstudied updo.

At-home: Brush hair forward to create lift at the crown; then comb hair back into place, making sure to smooth the sides into place using a natural bristle brush; curl the back using steam rollers or pin curls and a setting lotion; release and shape into an unstudied updo.

WELL ROUNDED: YOUR GREAT STYLE GLOSSARY

Putting your best look forward is a cinch when you have the right maintenance treats, tools, and tips. Here's a go-to list:

AID	BENEFIT	ON-POINT PICK
Hydrating Shampoo	cleanses, detangles, conditions	Design Essentials Moisture Retention Conditioning Shampoo
Moisturizing Conditioner	replenishes, repairs, maintains	Optimum Care Salon Collection Fortifying Conditioner
Protein Conditioner	revitalizes, strengthens, restores	PhytoSpecific Energizing Concentrate
Restructuring Conditioner	rebuilds damaged hair, nourishes	KMS California Moist Repair Restructuring Therapy
Hair Mask	hydrates, strengthens, smooths	Ojon Revitalizing 2-min Hair Mask
Leave-in Treatment	nourishes and fortifies	Infusium 23 Repair and Renew Leave-In Treatment
Daily Leave-in Conditioner	treats, hydrates, lubricates, and protects	Pantene Pro-V Relaxed & Natural Daily Oil Cream Moisturizer
Wrap/Setting Lotion	adds body, offers a smooth set or wrap, prevents frizzies	Creme of Nature Argan Oil Foaming Wrap Hair Lotion
Mousse	creates fullness, adds body, defines	Aveda Phomollient Styling Foam
Light Pomade	hydrates, lubricates, conditions, polishes	PhytoSpecific Nourishing Styling Cream
Hair Cream	replenishes, hydrates, add shine	SoftSheen-Carson Dark and Lovely Healthy-Gloss Moisture Hair Crème
Shine Serum	coats, adds sheen	Creme of Nature Argan Oil Gloss & Shine Polisher
Sheen Spray	adds a glossy sheen, protects	MoroccanOil Glimmer Shine Spray

Commander in Chic

AID	BENEFIT	ON-POINT PICK
Liquid Oils	renews, lubricates, seals moisture, and imparts shine	Moroccanoil Moroccan Oil
Heat Protectant	softens, improves straightening, buffs against heat	Kérastase Nutritive Nectar Thermique
Holding Spritz	keeps hair in place, imparts flexible hold	Motions Light Hold Working Spritz
Hairline control	smoothes, checks flyaways, holds	Organic Root Stimulator Olive Oil Edge Control
Volumizer	adds body	TRESemmé Big Boost Root Lift Spray
Extension Care	smooths, revitalizes, protects	Kimble Hair Care Systems Untangle the Shampoo and Untangle the Conditioner
Wide-tooth Comb	detangles	Denman Detangling Comb
Large-Tooth Styling Comb	mimics hand combing, defines layers	Gold Magic Fluff Comb
Rat-Tail Comb	great for precise partings	Mason Pearson Rat Tail Comb
Paddle Brush	detangles, smooths	HairArt H3000 Tourmaline Paddle Brush
Natural Bristle Brush (pure boar bristles)	styles, smooths	Denman 8 Row Styling Brush
Blow-Dryer & Comb Attachment	delivers a silky, smooth finish	Tourmaline Tools 1875W Tourmaline Ionic Professional Dryer
Flat Iron	gives a smooth, sleek finish	BaByliss Pro Nano Titanium Ultra Flat Iron 1″
Large-Barrel Curling Iron	smooths cuticle, delivers large curls	Gold 'N Hot Smart Heat Professional Curling Iron
Root Smoother	quick and effective straightening for roots and edges	R Session Tools R-733RC Root Control ½″ Barrel and Pressing Comb Duo
Large Steam Rollers	create shape and volume	Conair Curlcare Hot Rollers Hot Curlers w/ Steam Option

FRINGE BENEFITS

When it comes to selecting hair extensions or a great wig, don't sweat it—options abound. Whether you're looking for a color or volume boost, a texture change, or a completely new do, finding your perfect match is about having a clear strategy *before* you hit the beauty supply store. To simplify your decision, schedule a consultation with your hairstylist. There, armed with an open mind and pictures of looks you love, talk over such important considerations as how much maintenance is involved in the look you desire, appropriate hair texture options, the condition of your own hair, and your lifestyle. If selecting hair for a weave, your goal is to choose a texture that matches your own, especially if you intend to incorporate your hairline or to add volume. Whether you choose Indian hair, which experts like Kim Kimble, hairstylist to Beyoncé and Mary J. Blige, prefer as it most mimics fine, relaxed hair, Brazilian, wavy or kinky, selecting the best human hair extensions for your desires will allow you a great array of style, texture, and shade options. When purchasing, it's always best to buy hair by the ounce; this way you're sure of quality control and when you need to refresh your look, you'll have hair on hand that matches your existing extensions. Once you've decided on your style choice, let that guide the amount of hair you'll purchase. To keep your look salon-fresh, get a great cut, and choose products sans alcohol that will keep your extensions soft and lustrous as opposed to dull, dry, and brittle. Be sure to banish moisture-zapping cotton scarves and pillowcases from your collection altogether. And never leave extensions in too long—this is a road map to damage for your natural hair—therefore make certain to have your weave tightened every six to eight weeks. Extension styling does represent a commitment, but think of it this way: it's one that will allow you to rule your style day in and day out.

MIKKI-ISMS

Don't get stuck! If you're supporting your do with pieces, either use clip-ons or get the tracks you need as bonding always takes more than it gives.

Commander in Chic

On the other hand, if you're the experimental type and like to switch it up, then you're just the girl for a great wig. Think of this move as a simple one—with a dash of glamour—then work! A human hair wig is your best bet again, as they look far more natural, last well over a year with proper care, and offer you the kind of style versatility any great fashionista requires. However, if you're the sister for whom a wig is a great accessory, then go for a synthetic wig. Even though their longevity is in the "throwaway chic" category (they last only about a month), they do allow you to be as trendy as you want to be without breaking the bank. For certain, you'll want to have your hairstylist thin any wig that you purchase (as they all tend to be dense) and scissor it into a fresh cut that says "you." You'll also want to purchase a fishnet cap to wear under your wig to protect your hair from the wig's cap.

Finally, as tempting as it may seem, take care when looking to a lace-front wig. Unless you're a showbiz personality, this is not the move for you. Think about it: daily use of the glue could cost you your hairline. Not cool, so make the wise choice: style pretty and maintain the health of your hair.

MIKKI-ISMS

Your hair should be so fly that it looks as though you have a pro on speed dial.

MIKKI-ISMS

A saucy bang is always "in." Not ready to commit? Try a clip-in fringe. See hairconspiracy.com or call Kimble Hair Care Systems and Kimble Creations at 310.652.1822 to make it happen.

NATURAL GLAMOUR

The bob gets an injection of volume and style when worn au naturel. Here's what you need to know to turn it out:

Style Primer: Pro Tips on Working Great Style

Today's chicest bob styles translate to the most exquisite natural textures and looks—from Afroesque sets to braids, locks, twists, and beyond. What's key to achieving and maintaining a great look is the use of appropriate tools and stylers as directed by a pro to keep hair polished and prevent damage. According to Dickey, celebrity hairstylist and author of *Hair Rules! The Ultimate Haircare Guide for Women with Kinky, Curly or Wavy Hair*, your best bets lie in making sure that you find a care and styling regimen that is suitable for your texture, not someone else's. "It's about an approach to texture that is more customized," he says. Here, too, it's about incorporating those nurturing and protective measures that take into consideration your distinct care needs first and foremost. "Kinkier, curlier hair is a naturally drier texture," says Dickey, who has unlocked the mystery of textured hair to create iconic hair-

MIKKI-ISMS

Work it out. Don't even think about skipping exercise to preserve your hair—it shouldn't be an option. Rather, establish a regime and a coterie of looks that empower you to live your best life.

If you're working a "press and curl," go edgy and affect the illusion of thicker hair by playing your dark roots against a honey/amber blend of hues. After all, you don't have to stress the concerns associated with pairing a chemical relaxer and color, so rock.

styles for designers, advertisers, photographers, and celebrities alike, as well as a product line and a salon called Hair Rules.

This translates into a need for hydration every step of the way, from the cleansing and conditioning phase to the stylers. To begin, he advocates cream shampoos that are nonsudsing as they remove dirt and oil without stripping the hair of moisture. "Unfortunately, women are looking for miracles from their conditioner due to the damage caused by their shampoo, but there's limited capability of what a conditioner can do if your shampoo is drying your hair out," Dickey concludes. A leave-in conditioner that acts as a barrier for heat "similar to using a moisturizer before makeup," he adds, is key. Not to be left out of the picture is scalp care. Experts agree that your scalp is an extension of your skin and should be treated as such. "Good hair care is also good skin care. If your skin is naturally drier, your scalp will be naturally dryer, too," the stylist says. Pomades, waxes, and scalp foods can merely mask a problem and may even cause an allergic reaction as they sit on the skin. Dickey advocates nourishing essential oils. He encourages sisters to take advantage of these oils' therapeutic properties that nurture, normalize, and alleviate scalp issues. He recommends such oils as tea tree oil with its antiseptic properties and sage, basil, even pure aloe vera, which is naturally soothing and hydrating. Dickey's commandments for great natural bobs are:

- Maintain a really sharp line but make small tweaks to your cut: "Try adding a few layers so you get more versatility."

- Take a gentler approach to straightening: "You can have the same classic bob look by using a comb attachment with your blow dryer; it's about gently detangling hair that is naturally drier, so that flat ironing [and any heat styling] becomes less damaging."

- Mix up your style approach: "Try using a curl definer and wearing it natural; consider protective styles like twists—two-strand twists, flat twists—but always pretreat the hair before you twist. You're putting the hair away for five to ten days and if you're not mindful of this, then you're not caring for your hair." Rod sets or a straw set using a nice moisturizing gel or hydrating cream are also great alternatives. "Kinky curly hair has more pliability and you can do a lot more things under a hooded dryer than you could if you didn't have natural hair—it's about treating hair like a cashmere sweater—not a tee-shirt—and using tools with a purpose."

If your style is supported by extensions, it's essential that you protect the health of your natural hair by not weighing it down with too much added hair, which will weaken your strands and cause breakage or hair loss. Whether you choose synthetic or natural hair, what's important is not to leave in the extensions too long. If you wear braids, Dickey says, "Be mindful that they are friendly to your scalp and hairline, and again aren't left in too long." It is advised that you remove synthetic extensions (which zap moisture from your natural hair) within four to six weeks and human hair extensions every six to eight weeks and have your hair deep-conditioned in the process.

KEY EXTRAS: PRODUCT ESSENTIALS THAT GO THE DISTANCE

Depending on the texture of your natural hair and how you work your bob, a coterie of great care and styling aids is essential. Here's what should be on your checkout list:

AID	BENEFIT	ON-POINT PICK
Cream Shampoo	to gently cleanse without stripping	Hair Rules Daily Cleansing Cream
Conditioner	to condition, define, and elongate your natural curl pattern	Miss Jessie's Curly Pudding
Leave-in Conditioner	treats, lubricates, and imparts moisture	Avlon KeraCare Textures Leave-in Conditioner
Gel	smooths, creates hold, hydrates	Smooth 'N Shine Polishing Super Shine Conditioning Gel
Hair Butter	molds, sculpts, nourishes	Jane Carter Solution Twist & Lock
Liquid Oil	nourishes and treats	Pooka Pure & Simple Nectar Hair Oil & Treatment
Curl Definer	intensifies curls, defrizzes, heightens shine	Aveda Be Curly Curl Enhancer
Heat-Protectant	softens, protects, and resists humidity	Joico Silk Result Straight Smoother Blow Dry Crème
Sheen Spray	adds a glossy sheen, protects	Design Essentials Reflection Liquid Shine

Command Performance

When it comes to tools and stylers, here's what should be on your hot list to help you achieve the chicest styles.

1. **Wide-tooth comb for detangling**

2. **Blow-dryer** with a comb attachment to gently detangle hair while drying; keep in mind hair that's been cleansed gently and moisturized will blow out easier

3. **Diffuser attachment** to maintain great curl

4. **Portable hooded dryer** for great sets

5. **Tiny-barrel curling iron** to add more definition to your kinky/curly hair

6. **Flexible setting rods** (bendy rods) are super easy for creating a look—they're soft and go hand in hand with a hooded dryer.

7. **Tiny perm rods** are great for the ends of two-strand twists or flat twists

8. **Large hot rollers,** which are perfect for adding volume to fine, curly hair

MIKKI-ISMS

Hair tools aren't only **"accessories to great style,"** *they're investment pieces. For the sake of your hair's health,* don't skimp!

7

FACE FORWARD

When it comes to her beauty, Michelle Obama embraces a look we all can relate to—soft, polished, and impeccably glamorous. What I love most about her approach to makeup is that she never appears as if she tried too hard, a real no-no for any modern-day beauty. Certainly her well-groomed brows, radiant skin, and striking eyes make a statement all their own, but what also goes over big in my book as a beauty maven is her ability to style without looking overdone, even for those big nights on the town. For certain, these days the First Lady has a fabulous makeup artist at the ready to help her serve great face every time she steps before the public. However, what I know to be true from the moment I became a fan is that even as a young senator's wife, Mrs. O knew her face well and always looked effortlessly fabulous.

I remember the first day I met her back in 2006. It was on a photo session for the Thirty-sixth Anniversary issue of *Essence*, and I was so impressed. She arrived ready for her close-up, hair chicly styled and make-up flawless. Now I wish I could say that about every woman I welcome to the studio, but that's a subject for another time. Looking back, I can say that her trademark "power look"—based on high-impact neutrals for eyes, lips, and cheeks as opposed to full-on color (which when worn all at once can date most anyone but young models in print and on the runway)—was just as "brillz" then as it is now. This formula is not only a no-brainer for her multidimensional lifestyle, but also for her colorful wardrobe, since it guarantees that she never has to think about how her makeup looks with what she's wearing. This is a great approach for any busy sister on the move.

Though our lives may not mirror Obama's, we're all living a multidimensional life at this point in our history. We're busy moms, wives, career women, community saviors, caretakers, and more. All this requires us to look like the "Commander-in-Chic" of our lives, right? Who has time to figure out if her makeup works *with* or *against* her fashion choices? Like many of you, I have limited time to get ready—no matter when or where I'm going—yet I know there's not a moment when we'll accept looking less than fabulous! What we want is to do so *simply* and *well*, which is why I love a sister who plays a timeless formula and yet makes it look fresh and modern every time.

Take Mrs. O's daytime look, which is based on her passion for neutrals. This philosophy can work for anyone, whether your style is "classic," "bohemian," or "next-setter." Neutrals work across the board as a wonderful foundation for you to experiment with, for ultimately, it's all about selecting the proper tones and textures to express a look that says "you." Brown-sugar hues, as I've come to refer to them, needn't be boring. With today's technology, there's a plethora of shades in store that are sister-friendly and fashionably fab. What's necessary is establishing the look(s) you want to achieve long before you ever hit the cosmetics counter and then making the right choices from a palette that allows you the versatility you desire. Also important to working these hues with aplomb is setting them off with the right canvas—those bare essentials of concealer, foundation, and powder

Commander in Chic

that when chosen well look like *you*—only better. I've worked with many makeup artists, including Derrick Rutledge who keeps Obama's makeup pretty and polished, and no matter what look they're creating, they all place a particular emphasis on perfecting the canvas first and foremost, before ever applying a sweep of shadow.

For Mrs. O, Rutledge delivers a flawless finish—one that can hold up to the lights, camera, and all the action incurred in her workday. One application trick he relies on in creating a look that lasts for Obama as well as Oprah Winfrey (who graciously shares him with the First Lady), is firmly setting foundation in place with loose powder. "Once I've based the skin, I dip a latex sponge into loose powder, pat the excess off on a tissue, and press it onto the skin, beginning at the hairline and working in to the center of the face," as doing so seals the foundation, he says. Rutledge felt so strongly about having a base that was not only perfect for women of color and our various skin tones, but made sense via a long-wearing, shine-resistant formula, he created it. His

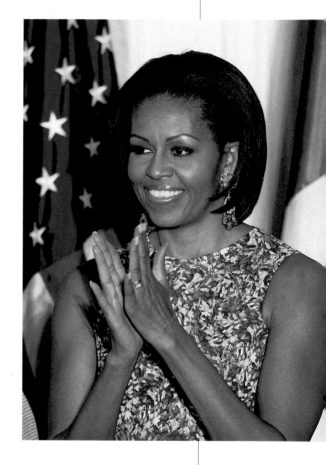

mineral-based foundation formulations (U/ooh/Cosmetics) can be used wet or dry as a base, and his cream compacts, which eliminate the need for concealers, as well as his moisture-proof pressed powders, are exactly what keeps a look "on." I've always said it's the canvas that helps to establish the "persona" of a look—whether healthy and sensuous, glamorous, edgy, or otherwise so this is where you want to place your focus, whether you wear makeup every day or not, because when you do, you want only the best at your fingertips.

Celebrity makeup artist Sam Fine says one of the major mistakes women make in basing their canvas is not applying the proper amount of makeup. "My new adage is 'more can look like less when applied strategically,'" says Fine, who believes that foundation gives you the opportunity to make everything else lay seamlessly. "Base products are meant to be worn together," he adds. So when enhancing your canvas, think in terms of layers: apply the proper amount of foundation for the coverage you desire, use enough concealer to hide imperfections, and finish with powder to set the look in place, as these base treats are designed to be used together. Fine compares this approach to the wearing of a little black dress: "You don't just put on a black dress—you put on a bra and panties or Spanx, et cetera, as they're the products that base everything else," he concludes.

MIKKI-ISMS

Do keep your makeup *fresh by using blotters* *for touch-ups instead of* *"re-apping" pressed* *powder—it's so over* *and* done!

Once you've got your base strokes in place, it's simply about knowing just how creative you want to be! Obama takes it forward at night where she's known to work a smoky eye in sheer grays (which I consider neutral territory for us) and woody browns to frame her gorgeous eyes. The look is always set to captivate with inky black eyeliner and a wispy lash, and I just love her for it. She is so fierce in her confidence to try new looks, and I say, why not? At the end of the day, soap and water takes it all off and, like Michelle, you're on to new ways to express what you so love about your beauty.

DEFINING A LOOK

Bare Essentials: The Perfect Base Is Your Best Backdrop

Every sister desires an immaculate, skinlike finish when it comes to "foundation"—those all-important base aids of makeup: foundation, concealer, and powder. We so dislike artifice and so the first requirement of a "perfect foundation"—which I categorize as anything that lies on your skin and sets the tone for your look—is that it be seemingly invisible, that it not camouflage the nuances of what we love about our skin or leave us with a masklike coverage that's totally unnatural. Thankfully, technology is speaking to us, including those of us on the chocolate end of the spectrum like Michelle, and so we need not be left out of the picture when it comes to natural-looking product choices. What's great now is that we too have the accents to play up our skin by way of bronzers that are rich in hue and highlighters that don't look ashy. Now we can mix it up and move through an array of finishes in base treats that allow us to look au naturel on the weekend, polished and finished at work, and utterly glam by night. Now there's a real definition of owning your look!

PRIME TIME

One of the important keys to looking flawless when it comes to makeup is perfecting the skin's surface *before* you apply your foundation. Nothing does this more effectively than a makeup primer that prepares your canvas much like an artist prepares her canvas before she begins to paint. Primers not only allow your makeup to go on easily and evenly, but make your skin appear so smooth. Worn over your moisturizer, primers are like the Spanx of beauty in that they diminish characteristics that you don't necessarily love, like uneven texture concerns and fine lines. It also makes your makeup last longer, helps to prevent creasing and, most of all, is cost effective as you'll use less makeup when you apply a primer first. Primers are available in formulas for face, eyes, and lips. And, adds makeup artist Sam Fine, "They're clear, so it's one size fits all." Now that's a real bonus!

Chart Your Course

Given the array of choices in makeup today, choosing the right base aids can be overwhelming to say the least. Here's what you should know when facing the counters and aisles in order to leave with the prime selects.

PRODUCT	FORMULATION	BENEFIT
Foundation	Tinted moisturizer	Sheer, skinlike finish with minimum coverage and a hint of color; great for those times when you simply want a skin-perfect finish
	Liquid	Offers sheer to medium coverage; oil-free formulas are best for oily and combination skin types; water-based or those identified as "hydrating" or "moisturizing" formulas are best for normal to dry skin; available in both matte and dewy finishes as well as mineral formulas for those with sensitive skin
	Cream	Provides medium to maximum coverage; available in oil-free and moisturizing formulas, imparts a flawless, moist finish
	Cream-to-powder	Offers medium to full coverage that dries to a matte, powder finish; suitable for all skin types
	Mineral powder foundation	Gives a natural finish with light coverage; checks oil
	Stick	Most valuable player! Provides medium to full coverage; doubles as a concealer; gives a semi-matte finish; suitable for all skin types
Concealer	Cream	Offers full coverage
	Tube	Lightweight cream; provides medium coverage
	Wand	Lightweight, lotion-like texture; offers semi-sheer coverage
Powder	Pressed	Provides medium coverage; zaps shine
	Loose	Offers light coverage; sets foundation; zaps shine
Highlighter	Liquid, cream, or powder	Imparts radiance; great for adding a glow to a flat base, illuminating target areas and adding a healthy, sensuous finish to bare skin
Bronzer	Powder, liquid, or gel	Offers a warm, sun-kissed glow (available with or without a shimmer finish)

Commander in Chic

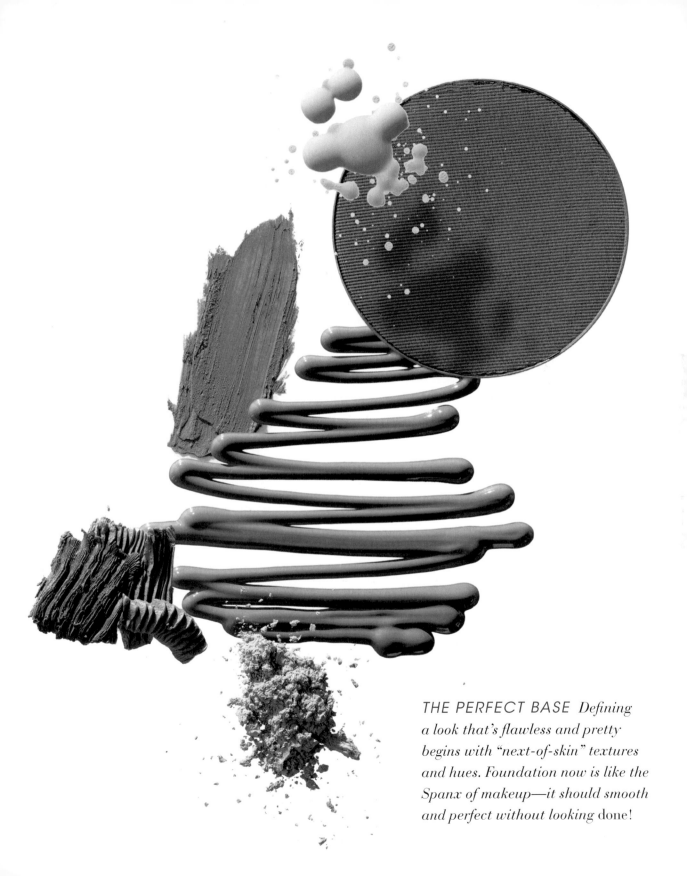

THE PERFECT BASE *Defining a look that's flawless and pretty begins with "next-of-skin" textures and hues. Foundation now is like the Spanx of makeup—it should smooth and perfect without looking* done!

CHEEK SHEET: A HINT OF COLOR IS YOUR BEST BALANCING ACT

The First Lady's sophisticated look always enhances what she naturally possesses, which is why *she* and not her makeup is always deemed as looking great. In truth, it's not about how we accentuate the makeup, but rather how well we accentuate *our* beauty. This is so important when it comes to using blush and highlighting your cheekbones. Like many experts, Fine believes that we have to redefine the way that we view blush, as we don't blush in the traditional sense. "It's no longer the '70s or the '80s when we knew blush to be the very red/burgundy standout shades offered to women of color," he says. And though blush is a minor player for us, it can make or break a look, so whether you prefer a cream, gel, or powder, know that application is everything and always aim for an effect that warms the cheeks and adds a little dimension (breaking up the flat finish that base and face powder alone can create)—nothing more.

Most experts follow a layering approach in that they use a brown-based hue first and then apply a light layer of color followed by a highlighter. To achieve your most seamless finish, smile and apply your chosen hue or hues sparingly from the apples of your cheeks up toward your hairline, until you reach your desired tone. Follow by applying a sweep of highlighter along the cheekbone to bring a soft glow to the skin.

MIKKI-ISMS

Never, ever match your makeup to your clothes. Makeup should complement, not match. Besides, you're far more creative than that—right?

Commander in Chic

What also ensures a natural finish is good lighting. I find daylight the most accurate, so I've placed my vanity right in front of the window in my bedroom. Having a vanity allows me to sit and look Ms. Mikki squarely in the face and get it right every time! I really think applying your makeup while seated at a vanity is so relaxing, as it keeps you from being in a hurry with yourself. Lord knows we move at a sprinter's pace day in and day out, so having this little time for self should be an essential way to begin your day. It's so much better than standing over your bathroom sink or doing your makeup behind the wheel. You deserve so much more than that. Think of finding a vanity or a small table and a charming chair and let it be a great excuse to go antique-ing! In the meantime, try placing your mirror on a windowsill—it will guarantee a look that's totally flattering.

Cheek to Chic

Blush 101

Cheek shaping can be fresh and easy when you understand which textures and tones work best for you. By far, powder blush is the easiest to apply, followed by cream formulations, which blend so well you can use your fingers or a latex wedge to achieve your desired amount of color. Gel sticks can be applied directly to the skin and feathered using a latex sponge for a soft, natural wash of color. Keep in mind that given technological advances in makeup, it's easy to use nontraditional products to add color to your cheeks as well. For example, many makeup artists use pigments or shadows from popular cosmetic companies like M.A.C. and Makeup Forever to achieve the look they desire, especially on women of color. Imagine what it's like if you're a sister who's on the fair end of the color zone trying to find a toasty peach- or salmon-hued blusher that has just the right amount of depth, plus color, minus the ash. Ditto if you're a sister with a rich brown

CHEEK TO CHIC

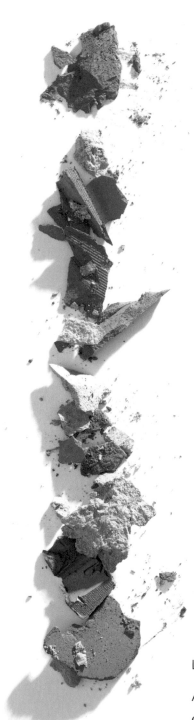

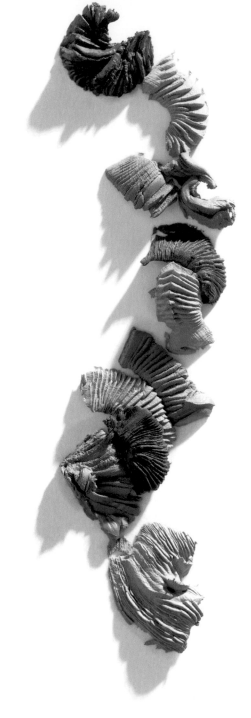

LEFT *Powder: delivers a soft, matte film of color*

ABOVE *Cream (pot or stick): imparts subtle color with a moist finish*

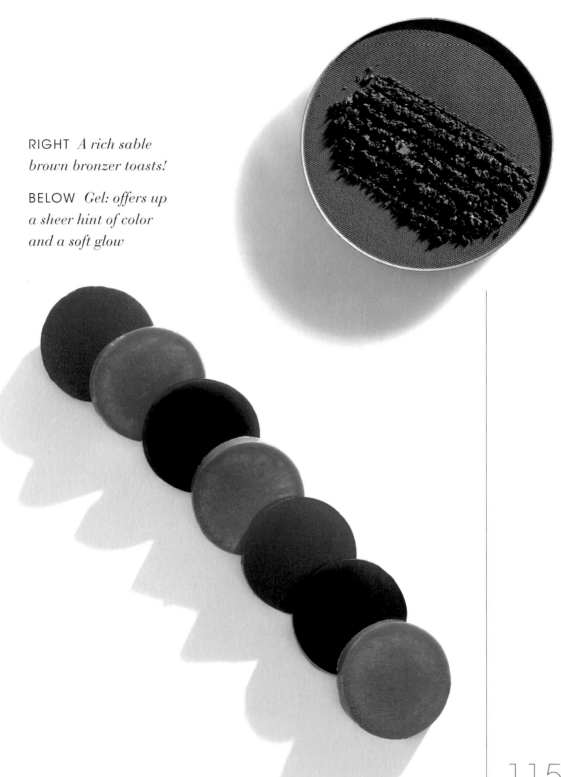

RIGHT *A rich sable brown bronzer toasts!*

BELOW *Gel: offers up a sheer hint of color and a soft glow* complexion in search of a cinnamon- or sable-hued blusher in a creamy formula that will look natural on you. In both cases it's about finding the product that helps you achieve the look you want, and that might mean using products and formulations that help you do so from a category other than those identified as "blush." Personally, I love orange hues as they work well with my rich brown skin, and so I'm always on the beauty prowl for those that work according to the season. In summer I'm reaching for those with hints of sunny gold; in winter it's about those that are browned or toasted—that echo my natural hues. Whether they are actual blushers or cream shadows or bronzing powders doesn't matter as they help me work a look. Again, thanks to modern technology, they go on well and last. So be sure to keep an open mind and remember it's all about you and the look that you want to achieve.

SHEER GENIUS

Finding your most natural cheek tones is as simple as shopping with your skin's undertone in mind.

Yellow-orange undertones: Yellow or warm blush shades (peach, orange, terracotta)

Red-orange undertones: Warm blush shades (single or multihued blush/bronzer/highlighters, cinnamon browns; these hues will ensure that you don't add more red tones to your skin)

Blue-red undertones: Cool or blue-based blush shades coupled with rich browns (browned roses, browned berries, layered over sable browns)

EYE STYLE: WORK A CAPSULIZED COLLECTION OF SOPHISTICATED BASICS FOR A STATEMENT-MAKING LOOK

Like most sophisticates, Mrs. O's eye style reflects a palette of precise neutrals, from soft pales to smoky deeps, along with liner treatments and flirty faux lashes. She's also keen on those deftly arched brows that really punctuate her look. To me, brows are the hood of the face as they really frame your look. In fact, many makeup artists set the brows in place first, *before* applying eye shadow, as it's an important part of the eye space and, again, really defines your look. I find when I do so, it really causes me to use my eye accents of shadow, liner, and mascara differently, and I'm far more creative at making a statement that's distinctly mine. For sure, "making eyes" is really a fabulous form of expression and one of the most fun ways to create a look using makeup like a painter's palette. Every time I see Mrs. O, I find that though her eyes are always creatively chic, the palette doesn't vary. The "look" sticks to smart hues and techniques that bring her eyes into focus. Why not create your own capsulized collection of smart picks that allow you to create a dazzling array of looks in no time? It's so savvy and far less costly than buying a zillion different products that take up more storage space than you should ever allow. I think every chic-ster should know how to play variations on a signature theme that works. Through the "Obama lens"—here are three eye-catching takes on style and a coterie of minimalist accents to get you there.

EYE SCOOP

Daytime Ease

Capture the Look. Polished nudes with a bit of depth define eyes in seconds. Work a sweep of a cool brown shadow on the lids and soft black eyeliner close to the root of the lashes for depth; finish with mascara, individual lashes (for additional thickness), and brow gel to set your frame in place.

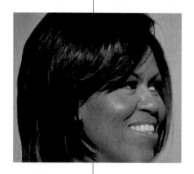

Eye Essentials: woodsy brown eyeshadow, black pencil eyeliner, volume-building mascara, individual lashes, brow gel

Chic Mystique

Capture the Look. Jet liner against earthy nudes give eyes a touch of sophistication without looking overdone. Make it happen with a potted gel or cream eyeliner in a rich black to fully frame eyes; set off by applying a sheer, muted brown shadow as a backdrop. Complete the look with wispy lashes and a few sweeps of a lengthening mascara. Define and fill your brows using a slanted brush and a brown brow powder (so the look stays soft and modern).

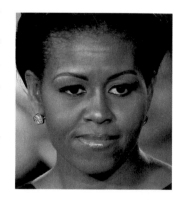

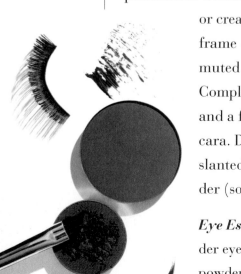

Eye Essentials: black gel or cream eyeliner, muted brown powder eyeshadow, lengthening mascara, wispy lashes, brown brow powder, slanted brush

Evening Cool

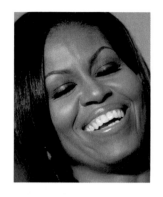

Capture the Look. Glittering nights call for provocative eyes. Ignite yours in inky-deep shadows in a mix of textures for layering from lid to crease, in shades of charcoal (softer than black) and an espresso brown. Apply the deeper hue close to your lashes and in the crease; place the lighter shade on the lid and blend, blend, blend to create a look that's sultry yet seamless. Using a fine liner brush and liquid eyeliner, work a fine, spidery sweep of liner from corner to corner. Finish by applying a pair of flirty lashes. Once dry, stroke on a few coats of mascara. Set the look by accentuating brows with a fine brow pencil.

Eye Essentials: deep brown powder eyeshadow, charcoal eye crayon, eyeliner brush, liquid eyeliner, fine brow pencil, mascara, full lashes

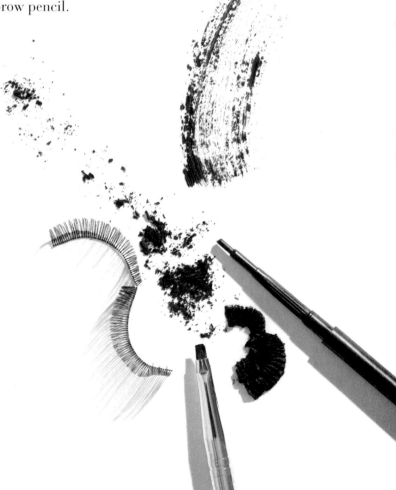

CHANGE AGENTS

When you've got great style makers at your fingertips, the possibilities are endless. Here's a roundup of the best picks—from nude hues for every skin tone to punctuating accents—to help you create your go-to stash.

Must-Haves

Nude Finds

1. Lancôme Color Design Eye Shadow in Waif

2. Bobbi Brown Eye Shadow in Tan

3. M.A.C. Cosmetics Eye Shadow in Cork

4. Chanel Ombre Essentielle Soft Touch Eyeshadow in Sand

5. Estée Lauder Pure Color Eye Shadow in Chocolate Bliss

6. Clinique Colour Surge Eye Shadow Stay Matte in Sable

7. M.A.C. Cosmetics Eye Shadow in Corduroy

8. Bobbi Brown Eye Shadow in Chocolate

9. Lancôme Color Design Eye Shadow in Faux Pas

10. M.A.C. Cosmetics Eye Shadow in Embark

11. Lancôme Color Design Eye Shadow in Matte

12. NARS Matte Eye Shadow in Coconut Grove

Liner Classics

1. Revlon ColorStay Liquid Eye Pen in Blackest Black

2. Make Up For Ever Aqua Eyes in Pearly Brown

3. Clinique Quickliner for Eyes Pencil in Slate

4. Bobbi Brown Long-Wear Gel Liner in Chocolate Shimmer Ink

Lash Support

1. Thickening: Diorshow Mascara

2. Lengthening: CoverGirl LashBlast Lengthening Mascara

3. Curling: Flirt It Curl Lash Curling Mascara

4. Tear-proof: Lancôme Hypnôse Waterproof Mascara

5. Sensitive Eyes: Almay One Coat Mascara

MIKKI-ISMS

Mix it up by working a sheer smoky eye from lid to crease in a supersexy tonal hue. Try mixing dark gray and beige or chocolate and bronze. How fab!

Don't be caught looking less than "code-chic!" *Groomed brows and lush lashes (real or faux) define a look in nano seconds.* Spring for it!

Faux Real

1. Wispy strip lash—great for day: Ja'Maal Buster eyelashes

2. Full strip lash—great for evening: M.A.C. Cosmetics 36 Lash

3. Individual lashes—single and cluster lashes, perfect for accenting outer corners, creating a lush look, most natural in appearance: Ardell Duralash Flare Short Black Individual Lashes

Brow Wonders

1. Pencil

2. Powder

3. Brow gel or clear gel mascara

MIKKI-ISMS

Dare to go bare: try a clean, retro-chic approach by playing a look based on flirty lashes, cream eyeliner, and a thicker brow against a matte nude lip. Terribly chic? Indeed.

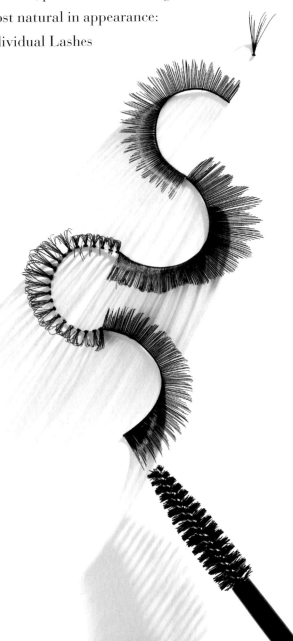

OVER THE TOP

A polished look always rests on how well one's brows are defined. Fabulously tended brows that bear no stray hairs that aren't overplucked or overarched convey a sense of confident, well-groomed style. To achieve your best look, I say consult a pro, at least to establish your ideal shape, since this is as important as any other beauty service. Think of it on par with seeing your hairstylist or colorist. Once your "perfect pair" has been set, then it's about maintenance, maintenance, maintenance. Here's what you need to know to stay in shape:

- Choose your hair removal method, taking into consideration the texture and thickness of your brow as well as your skin type. If your hair texture is coarse and your brows are thick, professional waxing might be best as tweezing may be unbearable. Waxing is also great for removing unwanted hair growth between your brows. If your hair is fine and you have minimal shaping to manage, tweezing is as simple as 1-2-3. If your skin is dry or sensitive, you'll find tweezing or threading your best bets.

- Before beginning your at-home maintenance process, make sure you have a great brow kit (see damoneroberts.com) or a brow brush, straight-edge cuticle scissors, and a sharp pair of tweezers on hand. Dull or poor-quality tweezers can cause hair to break as opposed to being lifted out squarely from the root.

- To begin, brush brows up and trim the long hairs that extend beyond your basic brow line. Comb hairs down and repeat. Next, gently pull your skin until it's taut and tweeze any stray hairs that fall below the brow bone, never on top, since doing so will distort your natural line. If you're sensitive to the "pain of the pluck," numb the area first with an ice cube or teething gel. Always grip individual hairs (never clusters or you'll be left with gaping holes in your brow—not good!) and remove in the same direction as the hair grows.

- To shape, fill in any sparse areas using a slanted brow brush and brow powder or a fine brow pencil in a shade that matches your brow color.

- Finally, comb through brows using a brow gel or for coarse hair a clear gel mascara to set the look.

LIP PARADE: A PALETTE OF CHIC, PARED-DOWN CLASSICS ADD POLISH AND PIZZAZZ

Timeless hues and modern textures come together to define and complete Michelle's beauty statement in a "less is more" take that always works. For the most part, she chooses a pretty deliberate formula: brown-based neutrals that look ultra-sophisticated and naturally glamorous. That's not to say she doesn't work the occasional browned rose or a browned red. After all, we know she loves to mix it up just like the rest of us. However, by and large, you can count on her to play a great nude to perfection.

MIKKI-ISMS

Do hit cosmetic counters that allow you to put together your own capsulized collection of hues in a single compact. Two hot to miss: Bobbi Brown and Trish McEvoy.

LIP LESSONS

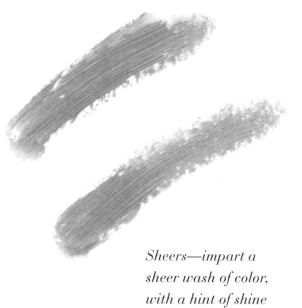

Matte—gives a non-shiny, full-coverage finish

Sheers—impart a sheer wash of color, with a hint of shine

Satin—offers a creamy, opaque finish

126 | *Commander in Chic*

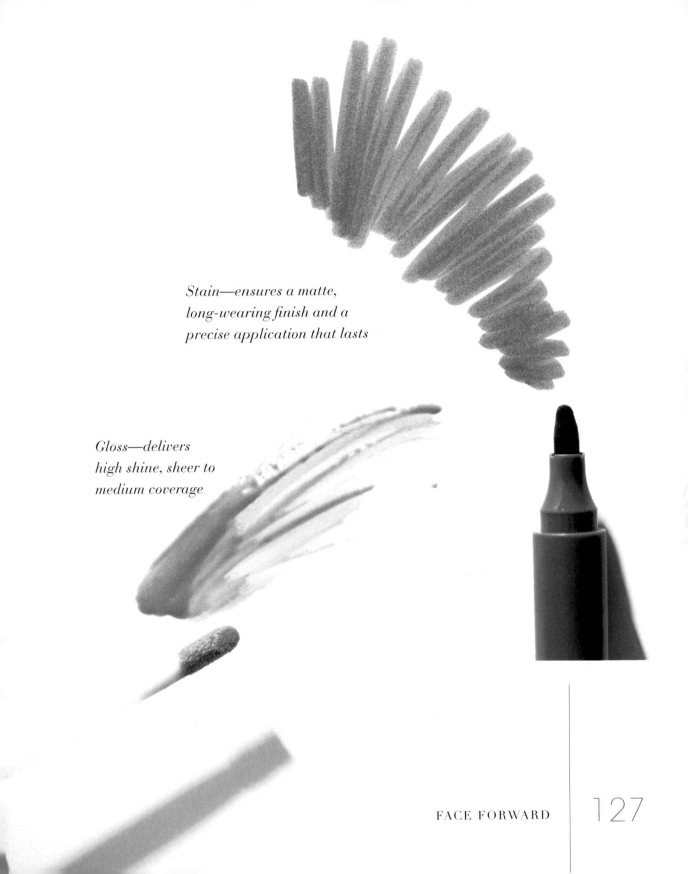

Stain—ensures a matte, long-wearing finish and a precise application that lasts

Gloss—delivers high shine, sheer to medium coverage

WORD OF MOUTH

Chic, sexy, and understated nude lips make the most modern impact next to red. However, only the smoothest lips need apply. Dry, cracked, or peeling lips are the "kiss of death" when it comes to working nude hues as tones like this showcase everything—including that which you'd like to conceal! To work your ultimate pout, give lips the same TLC that you give your facial skin with a regimen that refines, hydrates, and protects them year-round. Here's your how-to:

- **Buff:** Exfoliate lips regularly using a washcloth, a soft toothbrush, or creamy facial or lip exfoliant

- **Hydrate and Protect:** Moisturize lips throughout the day by wearing a hydrating lip balm or cream that contains an SPF under your lip color

MIKKI-ISMS

Be creative— find your best nude lip hue and glam it to the max! Gloss it, matte it, and by all means, gild it to perfection!

When wearing a nude lip, work it with effortless elan. Take a clean-glamour approach and aim for a fresh, sensuous finish by tapping on your lipstick with your ring finger or just applying a slip of a "sheer" or a gloss. If you choose a matte, apply with a lip brush and then blot. Don't stress it if your lips are somewhat uneven in tone, create the coverage you desire using a stick foundation, and complete the look by applying your lip color and carry on!

THE RIGHT BUFF

Mastering the art of successfully wearing nude lips can be tricky, but when you find the hues that work for you, it's just great. To avoid looking washed out, make sure your selects have a hint of color—from rosy flesh tones to those that are brick-oven warm, browned, and/or slightly sun-kissed. Keep in mind that it's important that the nude you choose never appear dry or flat (like foundation), as it'll be certain to make you look washed out. According to Fine, to get dimension, which is key, "You have to add punch. For example, a little caramel or rose to it or an undertone that boosts so it's a little more than nude." Fine also favors a light layer of gloss, which also adds dimension, shine, and separates it in texture from the skin, which is naturally more matte. Rutledge loves basing the lips with foundation first to add that extra layer for one's lip pencil and lipstick to adhere to, and then a slip of gloss. Clearly, it's about making the right base strokes in creating a look that lasts and then applying your perfect hue.

MIKKI-ISMS

*Whatever your **makeup budget**, know that there's no need to turn in your "**glam pass.**" Just grab a **cute, roomy tote** (we don't do plastic bags!) and hit the drugstore for performance-driven picks and **sister-friendly hues** that are so there.*

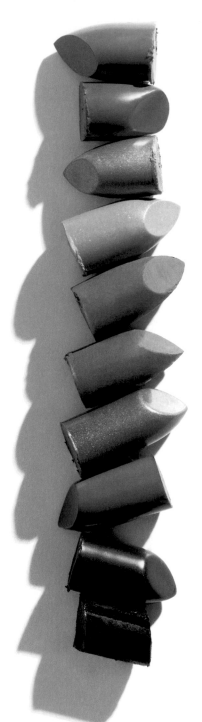

While specific makeup colors come and go, here's a capsulized collection of ready-to-wear shades to get you started on the best picks for your skin tone:

Lipsticks

1. Make Up for Ever Rouge Artist Intense MAT 1
2. Sonia Kashuk Lip Color in Truffle
3. Queen Collection in Cool Khaki
4. Revlon Matte Lipstick in Nude Attitude
5. L'Oréal Color Riche Lipstick in Toasted Almond
6. M.A.C. Cosmetics Satin lipstick in Cherish
7. Revlon Super Lustrous Lipstick in Pearl 305 High Beam Tan
8. Bobbi Brown Lip Color in Cocoa
9. Revlon Super Lustrous Creme Lipstick in Choco Liscious
10. Bobbi Brown Creamy Lip Color in Black Mahogany

Glosses

1. M.A.C. Cosmetics Lipglass in Shock-o-late
2. Bobbi Brown Rich Color Gloss in Merlot
3. Burberry Lip Gloss Mocha No. 12
4. Revlon Super Lustrous Lipgloss in Nude Lustre
5. Estée Lauder Lipgloss in Tempting Tearose
6. VMV Hypoallergenics The Big O! Glow Ultra Shine Lip Gloss in Honey Bunny

TIP BOX: EXTENDED PLAY

Lip liners are a real finishing product and instantly add glam and polish to any look. The problem is, they've gotten a bad rap. Far too often they've become the main event by being used improperly to visibly outline the lips, making a loud style statement all their own! The real purpose of a lip liner is to define your natural lip line and base the entire lip to prevent lipstick from bleeding. Contrary to popular belief, you do not need to buy lip pencils in the various shades of your lipstick. Simply choose a shade slightly deeper than the tone of your lips, and it will work across the board. A lip liner is an essential component of successfully working a nude lip look. "The biggest key that women of color need to understand is that there has to be something to define a nude lip, otherwise it will just be the color of your skin. When you look at celebs like Vanessa Williams, Queen Latifah, and others, they're wearing lip liner, which adds definition, which lip color alone will not," says Fine. He recommends choosing a hue that's one or two shades deeper than your skin tone. It will give you all the definition you need.

BEST TOOLS FOR A SPOTLIGHT-PERFECT FINISH

You can work a look with any brand of makeup you choose, but know that the right tools are essential. Think of them as your must-haves for branding your signature look. Those pictured represent my edits for getting started. As you move forward, add to your stash your specialty items that help you further define your style—at my last count I have eighteen natural hair brushes (synthetic brushes don't hold up or blend powders as well) that I would not be without and another ten at the ready, including miniatures for my clutches and touch-ups on the go. Here's a look at what should be on your checklist:

TOOL TIME Good-quality, hyper-fab, tools give you the most bang for your buck

Dual pencil sharpener: a go-to staple for large and small pencils

Eyelash curler: give lashes curl and lift; a real "bang for your buck" tool that gives any mascara more impact

Slanted tweezers: key for keeping brows and stray hairs in check

Latex sponges: great for cleanups, toning down makeup, and blending

Long sponge applicators or cotton swabs: for smudges and other cleanups

Twirl brush: for grooming brows

Slanted brow brush: great for filling in brows

Foundation brush: provides effortless application; allows you to control coverage and optimize blending

Powder brush: makes applying loose or pressed powder a seamless breeze

Blush brush: allows you to layer color easily and accurately without any harsh edges

Eyeliner brush: superb for rimming the eyes with wet or dry shadow, liquid liner

Eyeshadow brush: essential for quick and easy shadow application

Tapered blender brush: great for controlled shadow application and seamless blending

Retractable lip brush: for an even application of lipsticks and multipurpose creams

8

NAIL IT!

Obama's hands are always in the spotlight, as she uses them constantly as she speaks. I've always been impressed by how well-cared for they are, even before she became our First Lady. Mrs. O has always been a working girl, busy mom, and maintained a hectic pace long before she switched roles in service to the nation. But true to her style sensibility, she's always been clear about what works for her and wouldn't have had it any other way—then or now. In fact, I so love how she's nailed her current "classic and fresh" look by working modern nude hues on her fingertips that compliment her rich brown skin. And get this: although she has long nail beds, which allow her to work her short, squoval nail shape and not have it look hard or fake, working nudes gives her the illusion of long nails, as nude hues do for the hands what stilettos do for the legs! Need I say more?

What I also love about this smart and chic style choice is that nudes go the distance for us working girls in that they work with any wardrobe across the board, and when that inevitable chip occurs, it doesn't shout "I need a manicure!" As easy as this formula may seem, on the color front, not all nudes are created equal: some are cool, others are warm, some possess a yellow base, others a pink base, some are opaque, while others are sheer, and finally some formulas are shimmery, and others are matte. Finding your right nude is essential as every nude isn't a nude for the taking when it comes to women of color. For those of us with deeper skin tones, melanin often frames our cuticles and creates what appears as a dark shadow at the base of the nail bed. Aside from the overall skin tone of your hands as well as your undertone, this has everything to do with what nudes will work on you and those that will simply be out of the question. To quote my friend Mo'Nique, some nudes will make your hands "look like paws!" The Oscar-winning actress favors nude hues herself, both on TV and in real life, and works those that are light and warm as they compliment her beautiful brown skin and yellow undertones. To that end, she avoids anything with a pink base, since they're simply not flattering. When tipping a nude to a trendy look, she works those with a cool, gray-taupe base for contrast.

In truth, color trends come and go, but a strong style sensibility remains. I find that nude nails fall in this classic yet always fresh category. And if you're in this lane, knowing how to determine your best nude is key. Here's a briefer on how to face the shelves and come away with the right hue:

First, determine your undertone, which fall into one of the following categories and appropriate shades:

- Yellow-orange undertones: Light, warm hues

- Red-orange undertones: Light, cool hues

- Red undertones: Light to medium, cool hues

- Blue-red undertones: Light to medium, cool hues

Second, determine your desired finish:

- Sheer

- Opaque

- Shimmer

According to nail pros Ginger Johnson and Sara Liz Pickett, of Ginger + Liz Colour Collection, there are also hues that compliment all skin tones. "Taupes with a lavender base look great on all skin tones and are an alternative to the barely-there sheer pale pinks we usually turn to when seeking those shades we deem as 'office friendly,'" says Liz. Other nail lacquers that compliment brown skin tones fall into what is commonly referred to now as the greige category (shades in the gray-beige family), which represent a newer category of nudes. You can also customize a signature shade by layering your favorite nude with a sheer shimmer overlay or a matte top coat, which is utterly cool. Whatever nude you choose, know that taking ultimate care of your hands and nails through weekly manicures and an expert treatment routine will provide the best showcase.

MIKKI-ISMS

I love a little embellishment on the nails, but I do believe in the expression "a little goes a long way." Why not layer a copper or silver sheer lacquer over your favorite nude? It's an effortless move that looks utterly glamorous!

LASTING IMPRESSIONS

Self-nurturing is so important in this day and age where I find us giving so much of ourselves to everyone and everything. Just like the First Lady, we're on duty day in and day out, administering to our family and others, and without question, our hands, if not taken care of, will certainly confess our hard work in a way that's not as beautiful as the service we so lovingly give. On a beauty note, our hands suffer environmental aggression unlike any other part of the body simply because they're always exposed. As tough as our hands seem, the experts tell us that the skin is very fragile and thin, which is why it's often said you can tell a woman's age or her projected age just by looking at her hands. However, according to dermatologist Dr. Gary Goldfaden, who practices at Academy Dermatology in Hollywood, Florida, by incorporating a regimen that calls on "regular exfoliation, hydration, nutrients, and sun protection, one can keep one's hands looking supple, young, and free of hyperpigmented spots." Here's what you need to know to keep yours politically correct!

MIKKI-ISMS

Shop call: do get yourself several pair of gauntlet **rubber gloves** *and a few "deli-sheers" (those transparent gloves the servers in the deli department wear) so whether you're cleaning the house or prepping food, your* **nails** *are* **well protected.**

Commander in Chic

HANDS ON

Dry Skin

Exfoliate hands weekly with a creamy facial or hand scrub.

Use a hand cream that offers a "glovelike" protective barrier after every cleansing; look for those that contain dimethicone and glycerin (protectants), keratin and collagen (together they work to provide strength, flexibility, and resilience), and an SPF of 15 to protect against damaging sun rays and hyperpigmentation.

Dark, Rough Knuckles, Hyperpigmentation

Exfoliate hands weekly with a salt scrub.

Treat the back of hands before bed using a hand cream containing alpha hydroxy acids for smoothness and a fade cream containing hydroquinone to decrease hyperpigmentation. By day, be sure to use a hand cream with an SPF of 15 or above. If you find lightening this area proves tough, don't hesitate to see a dermatologist who can recommend a prescription-strength fade treatment like Tri-Luma, a cream that combines hydroquinone, a retinoid, and an anti-inflammatory. Retinoids work by speeding cell turnover and are a real boon to this fast-acting prescription.

Veins

For apparent veins, experts recommend sclerotherapy, a procedure that causes them to collapse over time (see chapter 9 for additional information). According to Goldfaden, the appearance of dark veins can also be diminished without surgery with the proper topical agents. "Using a moisturizer containing vitamin K and arnica can reduce the appearance and inflammation of visible dark veins over time," he says.

Cuticles

Treat this live tissue, which acts as a protectant from bacteria, with pampering care by massaging daily with a hydrating cuticle oil or jojoba or almond oil so it doesn't dry out and cause you to reach for the clippers!

Never cut your cuticles; it's best to let technology do the job of keeping them smooth and tight.

Use a glycolic treatment cream containing alpha hydroxy acids in between manicures to exfoliate the cuticles and prevent buildup.

Should your cuticles split or peel (a condition caused by dryness, cutting, or picking at the skin) look to vitamin E and tea tree oil for speedy healing. Massaging an antibiotic ointment on them at night and sleeping in cotton gloves will do the trick as well.

MIKKI-ISMS

While we're not getting any more hours a day, do make those that you've got count: apply a luxe **hand cream** *before putting on a pair of glamorous rubber gloves to* **do the dishes.** *The heat from the hot water will make the cream* **penetrate** *and make your hands look* **divine!**

FOR THE NUDE IN HUE

The best nudes are to your hands what fine lingerie is to your wardrobe in that the right choices make all the difference in the world. Whether your preference is an opaque cream, a soft sheer, or transparent shimmer, here's a coterie of hues that could be deemed "absolute perfection":

1. CND Nail Polish in Creamy Cameo

2. CND Nail Polish in Putty

3. CND Nail Polish in Cheeky

4. Ginger + Liz Nail Polish in Brown Sugar Baby

5. Essie Nail Polish in Rock Candy

6. China Glaze Nail Lacquer in Pelican Gray

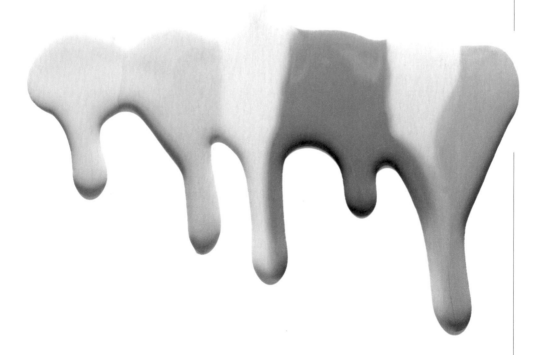

COVER YOUR BASES

Let's face it, a good manicure can be hard to keep unless you're working a perfect 10 via Minx applications (a flexible polymer film that shrink wraps to the nail) or committed to the upkeep of having your digits gelled over. If you're like me, however, and are working your natural nails, then you know maintenance, maintenance, maintenance is the order of the day. Over the years, I've always been on the lookout for that eureka info or product that will replace the basic upkeep with the miraculous answer. I have yet to discover it, but trust me, when I do, you'll be the first to know! I have learned that some practices we take for granted compromise our nails and the length of our manicure. Take, for example, having weekly water manicures, a real no-no, because in fact, water penetrates the nails and actually weakens them. It's something we don't think about, but in truth, it's the very reason we wear rubber gloves when washing dishes, right? So instead of soaking your nails in water during your manicure, try a warm hand cream or a hydrating oil soak instead. When I have my nails done, my technician heats a rich hand treatment in the microwave to soak my nails. It not only combats dryness, but it feels absolutely fabulous.

MIKKI-ISMS

Do give the French manicure a break. Why not try a half-moon look instead? It's so chic and unexpected. That's you, right?

Another culprit to great nails and long-lasting manicures is heavy-grit files (they act like sandpaper and wear nails down), so steer clear of them and always file in one direction. Another culprit is polish remover containing acetone, which is extremely drying. Remember: you want to protect your nails every step of the way, from start to finish.

To protect your nails and extend the life of your manicure, make sure nails are well coated, beginning with a base coat that's best for your nail type. For example, if your nails are weak and thin and regularly peel at a certain point, you should use a hardening/strengthening base coat. If your nails are hard and brittle and routinely break or chip, then you want to use a moisturizing coating to help with flexibility. You might also look for lotions containing alpha-acetoxy acid, which will also help prevent brittleness.

I've also found that touching up every couple of days with your top coat and paying special attention to the tips where polish normally chips will also make your manicure last, since this coating acts as a protective sealant against the elements. It also acts as a barrier against harsh chemicals like the alcohol found in many hair products (which is very drying), as well as soap and water and other environmental aggressors. But do avoid the use of quick-dry topcoats if at all possible. They shrink the polish as they dry and will cause polish to chip faster. Finally, take care not to use your nails as tools. Following these tips will go a long way in making sure your polish remains chip-free.

MIKKI-ISMS

What's utterly chic? A sandy nude nail topped off with a layer of sheer gold. How fab!

MIKKI-ISMS

I love a fabulous cocktail ring as a single statement on manicured hands. Don't know why the look is dubbed "cocktail"—fabulosity knows no hour.

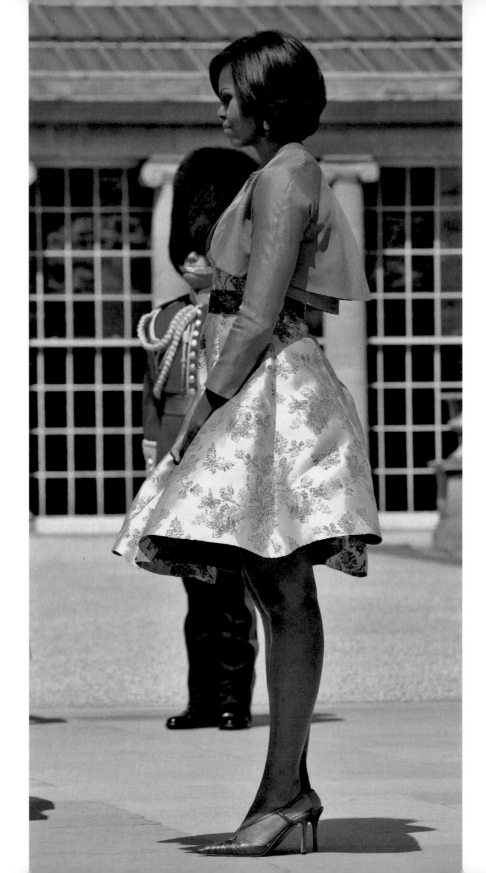

9

THE GAM SLAM

It's no secret: Mrs. O is not a hosiery fan. Given her dynamic legs and her passion for great dresses and pencil skirts, one can see why. Always true to form, you can count on the iconic First Lady to step into the spotlight with legs that are ultra-smooth, totally toned, and photo-op ready. Without a doubt, this is due to her diligent fitness routine and well-groomed approach to style. Like a lot of us, she loves pairing bare legs with a fab shoe—particularly a chic, polished pump or a smart flat. But don't let her choices fool you into thinking they're in the "basics category"—they're anything but! Take, for example, her wardrobe of pumps. She loves playing a little color against her rich chocolate skin. She also loves a great cut. Smart sisters like Mrs. O know that the most flattering pumps have a low, albeit sexy vamp, and those that showcase the cleavage of your toes have that essential "wow factor." In reality, this is such a leg-lengthening move, which is another reason why Obama's legs always look absolutely fabulous on-end, even when she's wearing a kitten heel. Let this be a word then to the well-heeled: it doesn't take a pair of sky-high stilettos to ensure your legs appear endlessly gorgeous! But fashion tricks aside, Obama's legs look just as fabulous in ballet flats—no easy feat, mind you. But like my personal trainer always says, Webster's is the only place where "success" comes before "work," and Obama works at delivering the "gam slam"! Rest assured, though, you too can bare it all quite beautifully with a simple strategy—starting now. Here then are your best moves to the prettiest legs ever—squats aside!

SATINIZE

Achieving satiny smooth skin is your first order of business for conversation-worthy legs year-round. The best way to turn them out is through regular exfoliation so you can defy ash and reveal the soft, smooth skin that lies beneath. Personally, I like a two-pronged approach, one that calls for a weekly manual exfoliation and incorporates the use of a sugar or salt scrub or a good loofah or skin brush coupled with the daily use of an over-the-counter or prescription-grade chemical exfoliant to really speed up cell turnover. Chemical exfoliants contain enzymes or glycolic or alpha hydroxy acids that slough off dead skin cells evenly. They're also a great precursor to any regime aimed at evening your skin tone. Enzymatic exfoliants are based on natural ingredients like papaya or pumpkin, which exfoliate without any degree of irritation in that they purely digest dead skin cells much like a scrub. Microdermabrasion also represents a fab option for ultra-smooth legs. This procedure, where a uniform spray of aluminum oxide crystals is administered to the skin and then lightly sucked away along with dead skin cells, is performed by both dermatologists and aestheticians. It's worth noting that the procedure you'll receive in a doctor's office will differ from that offered at a salon or spa in that the equipment available to doctors has more intense settings than that available to aestheticians.

THINK OUTSIDE THE BUFF

Enviable legs call for a velvety smoothness that's visible to the naked eye, and this clearly means that they must be fuzz- and stubble-free. For sure, shaving has its short-term merits—it not only removes unwanted hair but also exfoliates the skin in the process. At-home depilatories and waxing also represent good alternative methods for removing unwanted hair. So too does professional waxing. Like any removal process, though, all have their pros and cons. For example, we know shaving and stubble go hand in hand, especially for those with coarse hair. Ingrown hairs are a troublesome part of the process and, depending on your hair growth, repeating the process can be time consuming. Waxing and depilatories can cause irritation, and the challenge for us here is an increase of hyperpigmentation—not pretty!

Given today's technologically driven methods and products that not only remove unwanted hair but slow its growth, ultra-smooth skin long-term is where you'll want to focus your efforts. To this end, laser hair removal has advanced so far that even those of us with deeper-hued skin tones can now enjoy it. The process works by targeting the hair follicles, shrinking them over time through successive sessions and as a result, the hair that grows back becomes finer and finer until eventually the follicle is completely destroyed. The process also rules out the problem of ingrown hairs as the hair becomes so fine that it no longer turns back into the skin. According to experts such as Dr. Eliot F. Battle Jr., of Cultura

MIKKI-ISMS

Don't be a seasonal girl— *great legs* *call for a wardrobe of* *killer heels* *and* *flirtatious hemlines* *year around. What are you waiting for?*

Cosmetic Dermatology and Laser Center in Washington, DC, "When you combine the right laser with a practitioner who has expertise with lasers and understands the nuances of skin of color, laser hair removal is the best option to permanently remove unwanted hair." Coast-to-coast, the pros agree hands down that the safest laser for us is the Nd:YAG Laser, which uses a longer wavelength that targets the hair follicle without burning the skin. By and large, you'll want to see a dermatologist for this procedure and, again, one who not only has great expertise treating our skin but also addressing coarse hair, because the complications that can occur from seeing someone who is unskilled in this area are just too great. "When it comes to African American women, one of the big cons is having someone treat you who doesn't have the right equipment or who has the right equipment but doesn't work enough on skin of color to know how to adjust the settings," says Dr. Lisa R. Ginn, a board-certified dermatologist in Chevy Chase, Maryland. One of the biggest side effects of laser hair removal is getting burned and the resulting hyperpigmentation that leaves you with a series of tiger-like stripes all over your legs. "So you go from having hair that you wanted to get rid of to these hyperpigmented lines that are hard to clean up once they have set in," Ginn adds. Typically, one needs about eight treatments over the course of four to six weeks. And though it'll be a minute before you can toss your shaver, Dr. Ginn says, "The need to shave in between sessions should cease after the first two to three treatments."

Depending on the area being treated (full leg or lower leg) and the facility, average costs range from $650 to $900 per treatment for full legs and $400 to $500 for lower legs, per session.

MIKKI-ISMS

*They say **crossing your legs** is bad for circulation. Well, I guess circulation will have to **suffer!***

Another take on fuzz-free legs comes in the form of Vaniqa, a product that actually slows hair growth. According to Dr. Susan Evans, a celebrity dermatologist in Los Angeles, Vaniqa, though expensive, is effective. "It runs at least $100 when you use it twice a day," she says. However, Evans is quick to point out that it not only decreases the amount of hair, but makes the hair both finer and sparser in the process.

GET EVEN

Let's face it, attaining an even skin tone is a challenge for most sisters. There's no rhyme or reason to the way melanin asserts itself, which means any form of injury (insect bites, scrapes, etc.) or perceived injury (such as a repeated use, such as bending your knees) to the skin appears in unwanted areas of hyperpigmentation. This is especially true for those of us with deeper skin tones like Mrs. O. What's a sister to do? Get even, by arming herself with treatments that both banish discoloration as well as camouflage it so you can keep on stepping!

Today, natural lighteners such as kojic acid, arbutin, and licorice extract represent some of the options dermatologists use to help us achieve an even tone. However, treatment products containing 2 percent hydroquinone, the topical depigmenting agent that's been around for years and is contained in products like AMBI Fade Creams, are still at the helm. The latest findings, however, show that when combined with other treatment agents such as glycolic acid, hydroquinone not only fades darkened areas, but also helps accelerate the restoration of an even skin tone. The thinking behind this coupling speaks to what

> MIKKI-ISMS
> *High suede pumps in lipstick hues on bare brown skin? Now that's* sexy.

You want to stop traffic? Play a pencil skirt with a lacy slip peeking out underneath and a stiletto pump and know that you just might need a crossing guard.

many derms refer to as "combination therapy," a case where two treatments are more effective than one. In this case, the glycolic acid works to loosen surface skin cells and break down the barrier to hyperpigmented cells so the hydroquinone can impact them more effectively.

Areas where discoloration is resistant, such as on the knees and any areas where it goes beyond the skin's surface, will require a prescription-strength fade cream. Here too, many dermatologists incorporate the use of "combination therapies," where the use of a prescription-strength fade cream will be combined with a product containing alpha hydroxy acid or with in-office treatments such as a chemical peel or laser treatment to speed up the ultimate goal of an even skin tone. Again, it's essential that the clinician you choose is comfortable performing peels or laser treatments on skin of color, as burns can occur from both procedures. Chemical peels, whether calling on the use of glycolic, lactic, or salicylic acid, penetrate the top layer of skin and stimulate cell turnover. They're great for improving resistant areas such as the knees as, according to Battle, the darkening is almost always associated with thickened skin. "Alpha hydroxy and beta hydroxy (e.g., salicylic acid) peels can be quite helpful to both lighten the skin and reduce the thickness," he says. Average costs for chemical peels on the legs range from $200 to $400.

As with any procedure, there are pros and cons. The upside is a brightening of the skin and a marked improvement in texture. The downside:

if the discoloration is beneath the outer layer of the skin, the peel will not be able to address it. There's also the risk of further hyperpigmentation to any areas where the peel is applied if the skin is excessively irritated in the process. "Old dark spots on the legs are very stubborn," says Battle, and while topical methods will address surface areas of hyperpigmentation, lasers are the top-line choice because they go deeper and the treatments are spot-on. The process, when using the YAG laser, addresses our *deeper* pigmented areas most effectively. "If you've ever used a lightener on a dark spot, you'll notice that it will start to get lighter and then it just stops because the remaining color is sitting so deep in the skin that the topical can no longer get to it. That's where the laser comes in," says Dr. Ginn.

Once you're on the path to the flawless legs you desire, it is critical that you protect your investment every step of the way by using a good sunscreen with a minimum SPF of 30 *daily*—year round, as any sun exposure will only darken any discoloration, ultimately defeating your best efforts. Take heart, though. While you're in the "waiting zone" don't think that you have to reach for a pair of opaques or a pair of trousers! I have found that Dermablend Leg and Body Cover (dermablend.com) is absolutely fabulous at camouflaging discoloration. Trust me, it'll be your best kept secret, too!

MIKKI-ISMS

A nude high heel is such a fabulous way to extend your legs. Starting now, "make friends" with the salesperson at your favorite hot spot so she calls you when the sister-friendly hues arrive. After all, you know they are scarce.

GLOW FOR IT!

Don't get caught off-guard! When you're ready to go fully bare or wear a leg-revealing dress, having sallow legs isn't an option—not even in the depths of winter when everyone's legs can be a little lackluster. Incorporating a self-tanner will give you the sun-kissed legs of a vacation spent on an isle of your dreams. All skins respond to DHA, the active ingredient in self-tanners, and in a matter of hours, you'll notice your legs have taken on a bronzy hue. Thanks to modern technology, our options abound, from those products that are colorless to those that are tinted as well as tinted and shimmery golden for a rich, illuminating finish. When applying these products, always exfoliate the skin so the color will develop evenly and do look for those formulas that address your skin tone where applicable for the best results. Finally, always wash your hands immediately after applying so that the palms of your hands aren't bronzed in the process!

While at-home self-tanning products are great, nothing beats having a professional spray-tanning session. In less than ten minutes, a radiant, bronze hue is yours. What's also great is the ability with which the experts can sculpt your legs during the process and emphasize those assets you want to—like silhouetting your calf muscles—and camouflage those that you want to diminish, such as any pigmented areas. Yours truly is a devotee of self-tanners as well as a professional spray tan. What I love the most, aside from the quick and thorough process, is the

MIKKI-ISMS

Do remember that *fragrance rises,* *so don't forget to carry an exhilarating scent on your* *best dates* *and spritz now and again* *behind your knees.* *Need I say more?*

Commander in Chic

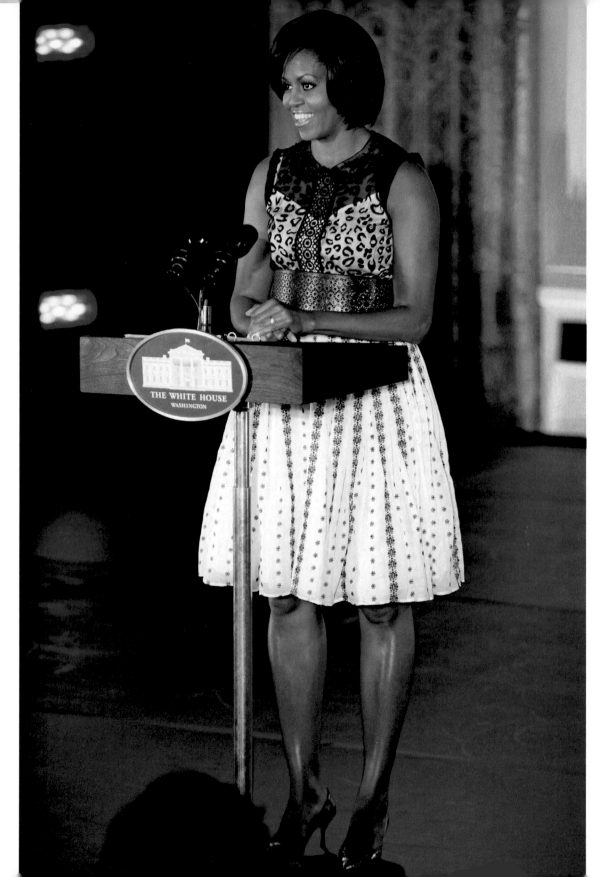

healthy bronze hue. I just don't like anything that shouts "fake," beyond faux fur and fabulous lashes, so it's essential that the results look natural.

When I'm in LA, I head to the Kinara Spa on Robertson Boulevard; at times, I also call on St. Tropez skin-finishing specialist Fiona Locke, who also sprays the celebs of *Dancing with the Stars* and others too fabulous to mention. All in all, you'd be surprised at the number of women who indulge themselves by applying a self-tanner or those who have it done professionally—from supermodels to top politicos. So I say, don't hesitate to get the flawless finish you desire by thinking the process doesn't apply to us sisters. You too can look "hotter than July" in minutes!

BANISH YOUR VEINS

Nothing kills a pair of picture perfect legs like spider veins. I say skip the "Mapquest look" and see a physician for a common procedure known as sclerotherapy, which banishes these unsightly veins in a matter of weeks. During the procedure, a saline or sugar solution is injected in the vein to destroy it, and the body absorbs the remains. Without question, this is the most effective treatment for spider veins and doesn't involve any more pain than the few pricks of the needle. Average cost for a session that will address multiple veins begins at approximately $350.

Commander in Chic

10

THE LAST WORD . . .

To one whom much is given, much is required.
—New Testament

I've had the opportunity to observe First Ladies and great ladies; I've worked with celebrities and so-called social swans. I've even met a renegade or two—you encounter all kinds on reality TV nowadays! Of all the women I've met, though, those who remain the most memorable have what I call *celebrité*: an undeniable mix of panache, grace, and spirit that makes them standouts.

Michelle Obama exudes celebrité, from her spirited attitude to the way she speaks, from the elegant and gracious way she carries herself to the élan she applies to everything she does. More often than not, we think it's the clothes that make the woman. Not so. I can't tell you how many times I've admired a fabulously turned-out woman only to have her open her mouth and crash it. Tsk! Tsk! What I've learned is this: part of looking pulled together is being together from *within*. Obama stepped to the top fully equipped to be there because long before she appeared on the main stage, she was clear, disciplined, and focused on *being* her best. When I speak of looking one's best and possessing great style, I don't simply mean from a fashion perspective. If that were the case, we'd all just go out and buy it, right? No. Any "commander in chic" knows that great style—style that not only impacts how you look, but also carries the kind of bravado that colors your world—is a reflection of the inner critical work one does to master every aspect of her life. Without question, great style is an inner and outer principle and ultimately it's more than the successful blending of a great personality and undisputable taste. It's about knowing your value and esteeming it with the highest regard because it has a direct impact on how you carry yourself, even when no one is watching.

When you know who you are—in other words "own your life from within"—then you can work it, and you don't need fashion labels because you're the real label. Or like I've said previously, you are the real "aspirational buy" that makes people sit up and take notice. This is what makes a woman memorable and interesting, that keen sense of awareness that makes her a standout. It certainly plays out in her conduct, for she's the one whose attitude is always both apropos and infectious. A woman with celebrité makes people feel comfortable and at ease. If she has a title, she doesn't wear it on her three-quarter sleeves. I so love that about Mrs. O. She's not only comfortable in her skin, but she'll make you comfortable in yours when you're in her presence because she's so *not* taken with herself. Who but Michelle Obama could touch the Queen of England and have her relax? This confidence of spirit allows you to stride through the world, take in what you need, contribute to making a difference, and yet never lose your pace on the way to your destiny. In the depths of your being, this acute sense of style makes all the difference as to whether you're on faith-forward or fast-forward, and know that there's a difference, for one is on purpose and the other is just "on," teetering on burnout.

I love how the Obamas have all their "style buttons" *on*, including the one marked "spirituality." It was encouraging to hear them talk to Barbara Walters about the value of faith in their lives. You can clearly see that they don't only have a "Sunday kind of love" (like the popular tune) with God. When we see them photographed heading to church, knowing that God is a regular counselor in their lives makes it truly meaningful. Michelle is quite vocal about their prayer life and her request to the Creator to "live long and strong," as she says. Given her actions in life, she's certainly supporting this ask on her part.

During my last visit to the White House, I had the joy of receiving my own private tour while I waited to begin the photo session with Michelle and her mom. I stopped to admire the images of the various First Ladies and the china each of them had chosen during her tenure. I had the joy of stepping into the florist quarters where the various arrangements seen throughout the White House are created. To my delight I got to see the expansive "cooler" (the size of a large room!) where the flowers are kept and get information on the various blooms, some of which were being used for an event taking place at the House that evening. I toured the halls bearing images of the Obamas at work and at play, saw the First Lady's Rose Garden, and more. And then I came to an area that stopped me in my tracks. It was an archway that bore not only the great carved ornamentation the House is full of, but the scorch marks from the great fire of 1814 at the hands of British soldiers. The fact that the House was restored by the original architect, using most of the carved though scorched ornamentation, stood as a metaphor for me. It spoke of resiliency, something a woman with celebrité has in abundance. I remember reading where Obama told Mrs. O and his staff that they must have thick skin for the journey on which they were about to embark in his run for the presidency and, sure enough, it was and still is essential for the road. Nevertheless, she has the kind of spiritual muscle that supports her no matter what the critics have to say. In our day-to-day, we must be the same and possess the kind of stamina that will take us the distance. Any time you step out for the greater good, you can expect to be tested. What's key is how you respond and what you take forward. Such is life. A woman to remember, though scorched sometimes along the way, picks up the pieces and not only rebuilds but also comes away better for it. And like any of her invest-ment pieces, she's resilient and ready to stand the test of time.

In the thirty years that I spent speaking on the pages of inspiration that is *Essence*, I've come to know a thing or two about us and what's important to the lives that we live. We're the nurturers; it's in our DNA. We give to a fault, sometimes to the point of having nothing left for our-selves. We come from a legacy that's loving and supportive. We stand on the backs of sisters who were both enslaved and free who nursed and nurtured babies who weren't their own. We've raised generations of fe-male youngins with celebrité. We work hard for every dollar earned and then twice as hard it's said for our psychic income on top of that. And yes, we love to style, and no one can like us. We keep people the world over watching to see our "next-ability," as my friend Macklin is fond of saying. Style is important to us; it's a form of self-expression, and we are masters at having our say. What we have to be about now, in the era of Michelle Obama and moving forward, is broadening our definition of what con-stitutes great style and being a woman to remember. As I put away my scented pen and focus my lens on the fabulous picture that we represent, here's the last word and then some to possessing great *style*.

Know your value. Your perception of who you are has a great influence on your emotional and spiritual well-being. Research has shown that we tend to act in harmony with what we perceive ourselves to be. This means that you're not going to live any better than you believe. This is why it's critical to possess a keen sense of self so that you'll see yourself as empowered and be in charge of every area of your life. Again, it's that sense of awareness that allows Obama to stand in uncharted territory and rule in the spot. On a lighter note, it's what allows her to repeat a great dress in front of the same crowd with great confidence. It's how she can travel the world over and never try to be anyone but herself.

Make room for your desires by thoroughly preparing yourself and, if necessary, taking the path less traveled to achieve them. Don't let anything stand in the way or compromise the quality of your life and those experiences you want to know.

Keep your head on straight. The Old Testament proverb puts it this way: "Keep thy heart with all diligence, for out of it are the issues of life." The directive is this: guard your mind with meticulous care, for it is the center from which your every action is directed! Remember: your purpose in life is altered only by the things you allow to have control over you and your perspective.

Be the gatekeeper of your "sacred space"—your mind. Think of your mind as your fertile garden—and know that the Word is "all things are possible to him that can believe." Be about the business of constantly pulling out any weeds of doubt, despair, and frustration as you seek to reach your goals and in turn fertilize this territory with seeds that will flower in your future with the success you deserve.

Live like there's no tomorrow! All women of substance do and because of this they're fascinating to be around, they're well-read, have a zest for life, are somewhat flirtatious, colorful, and well-traveled—even if only through their pages of inspiration—translation: the many books they've read! So live and make it count!

Take your cues from the right sources. Be discerning and take your prompts from the right people. It's about having those knowledge-able sister-friends to form your support network because supportive relationships promote your growth. Moreover, don't move through life acting in isolation, since it will often lead to anxiety and self-pity. Remember that it's important to be connected. Research has shown that when people are deprived of empowering relationships, they seek to fill that void—too often this space is filled with things that aren't edifying, that stunt one's growth, that compromise all one has worked for. From there it's a downward spiral that can bring about the wrong relationship with material things, people, food, and substances. So know it's important to walk with people who are smart, supportive, and have your best interests in mind. Never buy into the idea that it's "lonely at the top"—you can't use it. Mrs. O is at the top, and she certainly doesn't operate in isolation; she's got Barack and Mrs. Robinson and a host of others by her side, so take note.

Clear out the clutter. From the clothes you no longer wear and the things taking up space in your life and your home. That includes those vampire and toxic relationships that take more than they can give. Learn to accept that everyone isn't well enough to have a place in your life. I always say if you don't do "Judas" well—don't invite him or her to your table. As an added bonus, you'll be able to think and move clearly through life without these weights and have more of your own "aha moments!" instead of looking for them to come from someone else's untested wisdom.

Prioritize, prioritize, prioritize! Recognize that it's far better to give order to your energies by planning, rather than reacting to, what needs to be done. We must administer to ourselves and those we're responsible to and for with focus and the kind of organization that doesn't wear out our bodies and our minds. To be effective at our positions and good stewards of our abilities, we must use our energies wisely and prioritize how we spend them. When Mrs. O stepped into her role as the nation's First Lady, she made clear and distinct choices (for example, supporting military families and promoting good eating habits). She was intentional about where she wanted to make a difference. She also made her priorities known. Though she was the nation's First Lady, she was going to help her children with their homework, see them off to bed, and be a full-time mom-in-chief. Then she made sure she was up for the responsibility of all by *wisely* investing the kind of time and energy necessary to ensure she had the stamina to do so. So here are some pointers to checking yourself:

- Keep your goals realistic, start small, and continue to move. Martin Luther King Jr. said it best: "Take the first step in faith. You don't have to see the whole staircase. Just take the first step." Then as our mothers cautioned: "Don't bite off more than you can chew." In other words, pace yourself.

- Share your goals with your family and friends, so they can support you in your endeavors, which you'll need, as privately held goals are easy to lose sight of.

- Be willing to go the distance to reach your goals. Don't be a sprinter, be a long-distance runner. Remind yourself you're in this for the long haul, and remain committed.

- Learn to have a "hard out" even if you work at home. Don't be in bed Facebooking, tweeting, emailing and working into the night—you're better, smarter, savvier than that!

Invest in yourself. It's easy to lose sight of one's self in the busy-ness of life, and when we do, our best intentions go by the wayside. But I'm a firm believer that what you put in, you will get back. Get comfortable with putting the things that "move and improve you" on your schedule. No matter what season your life is in, now is the time to act with a sense of purpose and invest in your total "self," body, mind, and spirit. I've never seen a calendar with an entry called "someday." Many of us wait for it, but it just never comes.

Know that you must become your best advocate. Be the guardian of your goals. On a professional level, become your best marketer. Ask yourself what are you doing on a daily basis, a weekly basis, a monthly basis to empower the brand that is you. Where is your plan for mastering your life and reaching your objectives? How effective are you at networking and telling your story? What are you putting in place today that will help you show up ready to seize your dreams when opportunities present themselves? On a personal level, what's your health and "fit for life" plan? Who's on your temple management team? What skill set are you strengthening that will help you process stress in a way that adds to your growth? The wrap on this can be summed up in that old expression "take care of home first." Be reminded that it's not being self-centered, but self-nurturing. The experts say those with a high self-esteem and "can do" spirit gain their approval from within and not from outside sources.

Commune with your successes—not your challenges. The elders used to say, "Count your blessings"; in modern times analysts ask, "Is the glass half

Commander in Chic

full or half empty?" Don't own your challenges—they've only come for a season and one that will add to your growth, so pass through it and keep it moving. Don't keep company with your challenges, since anything you dwell on will take over. I don't know any successful people who got where they are without overcoming some serious challenges. Most of all, don't allow your circumstances or your "perceived circumstances" to rule your outlook and diminish your accomplishments. And here I say "perceived" because experts tell us that half the things we worry about never happen. I mean, we've lived a lifetime of tomorrows in exchange for so many "todays" that we've missed. Here's your best position: when challenge comes, run out to meet the hurdle and know that you're going to land a stronger person on the other side. We all know the biblical account of David and Goliath. The Word is that "David ran out to meet Goliath." Now notice that he didn't run *from* him. Goliath didn't have to find him or chase him down. David said, "Who is this?" David didn't commune with the threat that was Goliath. He was focused, at one mentally with the victory—so he showed up a conqueror, cut his challenge in more ways than one, and kept it moving!

Build your spiritual muscle. In other words, your resiliency, your ability to stand strong and handle adversity as opposed to letting it cripple you. To paraphrase Dr. Martin Luther King, Jr. who once said, "the ultimate measure of a woman is not where she stands in moments of comfort and convenience, but where she stands at times of challenge and controversy." It is in adversarial times that we grow the most. You know I've heard it said, "No test, no testimony." Things will come to test you in life, seemingly to see what you are made of. But this is where preparation meets opportunity. Tests come for a reason; they give you experience, build your patience, increase your wisdom, and, yes, they build your spiritual muscle. They teach you over time how to make the right response. So be

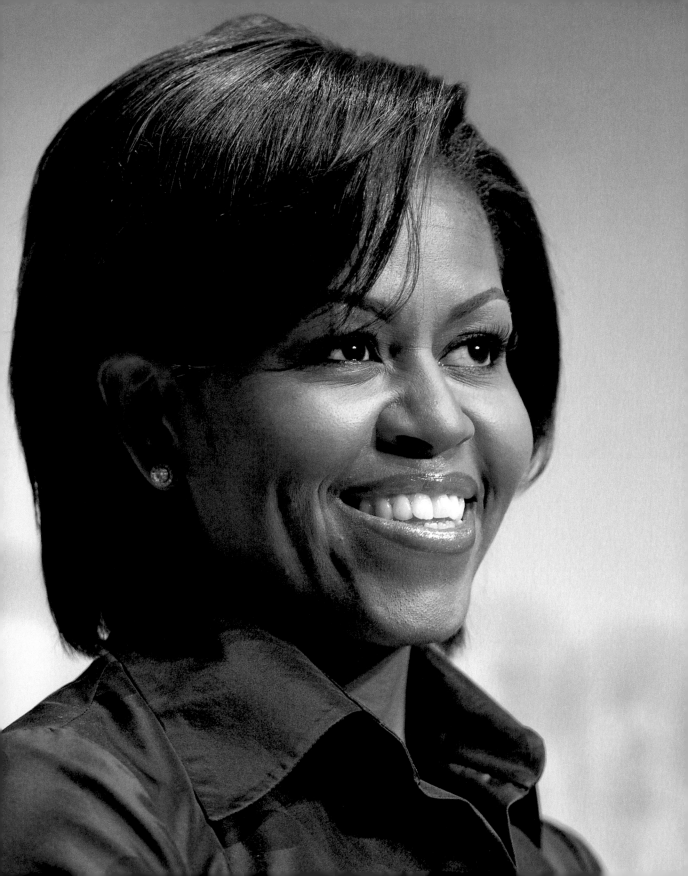

encouraged and know that the weights of life that you lift today will make you stronger for the positions and the times that lie ahead. Remember your job is to show up ready.

Don't let negativity get in your way! It's a deterrent that costs you time and energy. Every time someone or something presents itself in a way that causes you to think you can't move forward—refute it. Every "no" just means you have to be creative—not defeated. So put your blinders on and keep your inner dialogue on positive ground by speaking those things to yourself that will encourage you to get from where you are to where you want to be. Remember this: The Creator wants you to live an abundant life, not one crippled by fear, paralyzed by popular opinion, or drowned in negativity and self-pity. So whatever you have a tendency to succumb to—let it go! Write the message to yourself and hit "send."

A few years ago I had the extraordinary opportunity to teach at the Oprah Winfrey Leadership Academy in South Africa. And I have to tell you those young sisters ages twelve to fourteen blew me away! It didn't matter that they had come out of some of the most challenging circumstances one could imagine. What impressed me is how clear all of them were concerning their future. And I left there without a doubt that they would achieve their goals and become the leaders of the respective fields of their desires because they all carried themselves like they were already there! The Bible puts it this way: "Now faith is the substance of things hoped for, the evidence of things not seen." The key to mastering life, mastering challenges, and getting from where you are to where you want to be is faith. And you have to step out and keep going. You know with faith, you've got to do something—faith isn't just something you possess—it's something you act upon. Most journeys take twists and turns, you get breaks of straight paths, for certain you hit a few valleys, but if you walk by faith and not by sight, you get to the mountaintop. Through faith, today's thoughts and actions shape the future you want to know. On the move from where you are to where you want to be, make sure you keep your thoughts and actions faithful. Show up ready every day as the empowered woman that you are. Know that you can't be fearful and act courageous, so be fearless, aim high, and recognize that you deserve nothing short of the best and go for it! At the end of the day, that's what makes a real *Commander in Chic.*

ACKNOWLEDGMENTS

I Give Thanks . . .

To Almighty God who makes all things possible and through whom I live, move, and have my very being . . . my Lord and Savior Jesus Christ for His everlasting love.

For my mother, the late Modina Davis Watson, who taught me to fly and whose wisdom continues to steer me on the journey.

For Taylor, my darling husband, in whose unconditional love I am hopelessly lost and forever found.

For the jewels in my crown, my beautiful children, Samantha, Philip Jr., and Ms. Ashley, of whom I couldn't ever be more proud.

For my darling Princess, Modina—the sweetest grandbaby in a million—you rock!

For my family, whose love I am more than blessed to have—Daddy, my dear sisters, my brother, brothers-in-law, and countless cousins, nieces, and nephews.

And, for my brothers and sisters in Christ, friends, and colleagues whose encouragement and love I continually draw on.

And Praise . . .

To my literary agent Claudia Menza for the kind of encouragement that makes one fly!

To Judith Curr, for your never-ending support of yours truly and great enthusiasm for this project.

To my editor Malaika Adero for her priceless insights, sharp edits, and sweet inspirations —finally got my opportunity to work with the best!

To Soledad O'Brien, Kerry Washington, and Iman—my deepest gratitude to each of you for the "wonder" that you are and the treasured experience of having your support.

To the entire team at Atria Books who brought *Commander in Chic* to life, I bow.

To my art director Jason Snyder, whose visionary talent brought this book to life in ways that take my breath away.

To the one and only Tamara Houston, I'm honored and humbled every day to have you as a manager, let alone a friend. Hugs forever . . .

To my agent, Shelly Marchetti at APA—you rock and I love you for it. And my entire APA family.

To photographer Kwaku Alston—you're one in a million, and I'm so glad to watch your brilliance light up everything you touch. You're the "click," my Brother! Thanks for the cover image that says it all.

To photographer Timothy White, I couldn't admire you and your iconic gift more. Many thanks for the blessings from day 1.

To Gus Philippas, for your keen eye and always right-on-time style!

To photographer Monica Stevenson, for your masterful work and generous support of this project.

To my photo researcher and coordinator and dearest "BFF," Sandra Martin, for your unwavering support and excellence unequaled.

To Leslie Delavega—love you for your keen eye, wise counsel, and "spread the love" sensibility.

To my research team—Tasha Turner, Karen Good, and Bridgette Bartlett—for your attention to detail and support of this project. Know that I couldn't have done it without you. You rock!

To my *Essence* family, for the love and support of a lifetime! I couldn't have dreamt it better!

To Joseph Babineaux at Perspective Public Relations and Gilda Squire, Gilda Squire Media Relations, thrilled to have you in my life—you help me have a "say-so" in places I never dreamed. Here's to you, with hugs and love!

To Grada Fischer at the Fischer Ross Group, so glad to have you managing my purpose as a speaker.

To Susan Fales-Hill, for all that you are and for cheering me on with the kind of fighting spirit that continues to teach me to this day. You're one in a million!

To Monique A. Greenwood, for your sage advice and the ability to make me believe I can do anything!

To Sophia A. Nelson, for your edifying guidance, encouragement, and drive that continues to push me higher and higher.

To dear friend Pamela R. Macklin, for a love that's like "money in the bank"—it just grows and grows. Love you "Rexy"!

To Avis Yates Rivers, for all that you are and all that you bring. I just love you sis!

To the divine Ms. Harper—you're simply the best.

To all those who encouraged me to have a "say-so," I love you for this and so much more.

The many experts and companies whose time, vision, and insights will keep us all in the know!

PHOTOGRAPHY CREDITS

Page IV   ©Kwaku Alston/Corbis Outline

Page X   Photo by Alex Wong/Getty Images

Page XII   ESSENCE® used by permission of Essence Communications Inc., September 2008/Kwaku Alston

Page XIII ©Ron Sachs/Pool/cpn/Corbis

Page XVI   Photo by Jewel Samad/AFP/Getty Images

Page XX   ESSENCE® used by permission of Essence Communications Inc., May 2009/Timothy White

Page XXI   Photo by Gus Philippas

Page XXII Photo by Jonathan Ernst/Reuters

Page 6   ©Jonathan Ernst/Reuters/Corbis; Brendan Smialowski/Getty Images; Barcroft Media

Page 7   Photo by Saul Loeb/AFP/Getty Images; ©Marcelo Hernandez/dpa/Corbis; Kevin Mazur/WireImage for Time, Inc.

Page 10   ©Brooks Kraft/Corbis; photo by Michaela Feuerelova/isisfa/Getty Images; Dan Kitwood/Getty Images

Page 11   Photo by Eric Feferberg/AFP/Getty Images; Yves Forestier/Getty Images; Vladimer Rodionov/AFP/Getty Images

Page 14   Photo by Chip Somodevilla/Getty Images; ©Brooks Kraft/Corbis; Marcel Thomas/FilmMagic; ©Olivier Douliery/Pool/Corbis

Page 15   ©Joyce N. Boghosian/White House/Handout/CNP/Corbis; photo by Yuri
           Gripas/AFP/Getty Images; Pascal Le Segretain/Getty Images

Page 16   Photo by Marvin Joseph/*The Washington Post* via Getty Images

Page 18   Associated Press; ©Chuck Kennedy/White House/Handout/The White
           House/Corbis

Page 19   Photo by Dominic Lipinski/WPA Pool/Getty Images; Jewel Samad/AFP/
           Getty Images

Page 23   ©Jim Young/Reuters/Corbis; Pete Souza/The White House via Getty
           Images; Oliver Douliery/Pool/Getty Images

Page 26   Photo by Jim Watson/AFP/Getty Images; Jose Cabezas/AFP/Getty; images
           photo by Ron Sachs/Pool via Getty Images

Page 27   Photo by Mandel Ngan/AFP/Getty Images; Jewel Samad/AFP/Getty Images;
           Jewel Samad/AFP/Getty Images

Page 30   Photo by Associated Press

Page 34   Photo by Nicholas Kamm/AFP/Getty Images; David McNew/Getty Images;
           ©Alessia Pierdomenico/Reuters/Corbis

Page 35   Photo by Mandel Ngan/AFP/Getty Images; Brendan Smialowski/Getty
           Images

Page 38   Photo by Saul Loeb/AFP/Getty Images; Oliver Douliery/Pool/Getty Images;
           Carlos R. Alvarez/WireImage/Getty Images

Page 39   ©Eliana Apointe/Reuters/Corbis; Associated Press; Associated Press

Page 42   ©Miguel Angel Molina/cpa/Corbis; Win McNamee/Getty Images; Barcroft
           Media

Page 43   Photo by Saul Loeb/AFP/Getty Images; © Sabastiano Moreira/cpa/Corbis;
           Anwar Hussein/Getty Images

Page 50   Photo by Chip Somodevilla/Getty Images

Page 55   Photo by Alex Wong/Getty Images

Page 59   Photo by Mark Wilson/Getty Images

Page 70   Photo by Michal Cizek/Getty Images

Page 74   ©Samantha Appleton/White House/Handout/The White House/CNP/Corbis;
           ©Mike Nelson/cpa/Corbis; ©Larry Downing/Reuters/Corbis

Page 75   Lyle Ratiff/Reuters

Page 78   Photo by Prakash Singh/AFP/Getty Images; ©Samantha Appleton/White
           House/Handout/The White House/Corbis

Page 79   Jonathan Ernst/Reuters

Page 81   ©Kevin Lamarque/Reuters/Corbis; Jewel Samad/AFP/Getty Images; Associated Press

Page 90   Photo by Mark Wilson/Getty Images

Page 94   Associated Press; Tim Sloan/AFP/Getty Images

Page 95   Photo by Mark Wilson/Getty Images; Ron Sachs/Pool/Getty Images; Brendan Smialowski/Getty Images

Page 107   ©Olivier Douliery/Pool/Corbis

Page 111, 114–115   Still-life photography by Monica Stevenson

Page 118   Photo by Mandel Ngan/AFP/Getty Images; still-life photography by Monica Stevenson; ©Olivier Douliery/Pool/Corbis

Page 119   Photo by Ethan Miller/Getty Images; still-life photography by Monica Stevenson

Page 122–123, 126–27, 130   Still-life photography by Monica Stevenson

Page 131   Still-life photography by Monica Stevenson (makeup sponges by Mattesse; eyelash curler by M.A.C. Cosmetics; makeup brushes by M.A.C. Cosmetics; pencil sharpener by Sue Devitt; tweezers by Tweezerman)

Page 139   Still-life photography by Monica Stevenson

Page 142   Photo by Toby Melville/AFP/Getty Images

Page 151   Jonathan Ernst/Reuters

Page 162   Photo by Jewel Samad/AFP/Getty Images